Feminist P[...]
Perspectives from Africa and Beyond

edited by Rama Salla Dieng
and Andrea O'Reilly

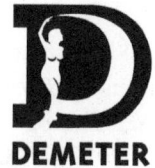

DEMETER

Feminist Parenting
Perspectives from Africa and Beyond
Edited by Rama Salla Dieng and Andrea O'Reilly

Copyright © 2020 Demeter Press

Individual copyright to their work is retained by the authors. All rights reserved. No part of this book may be reproduced or transmitted in any form by any means without permission in writing from the publisher.

Demeter Press
2546 10th Line
Bradford, Ontario
Canada, L3Z 3L3
Tel: 289-383-0134
Email: info@demeterpress.org
Website: www.demeterpress.org

Demeter Press logo based on the sculpture "Demeter" by Maria-Luise Bodirsky www.keramik-atelier.bodirsky.de

Printed and Bound in Canada

Front cover artwork: Serge Mienandi
Cover design and typesetting: Michelle Pirovich

Library and Archives Canada Cataloguing in Publication
Title: Feminist parenting: perspectives from Africa and beyond / Rama Salla Dieng and Andrea O'Reilly, editors.
Names: Dieng, Rama Salla, 1986- editor. | O'Reilly, Andrea, 1961- editor.
Description: Includes bibliographical references.
Identifiers: Canadiana 20200164147 | ISBN 9781772582284 (softcover)
Subjects: LCSH: Parenthood. | LCSH: Parenthood—Africa. | LCSH: Parenting. | LCSH: Parenting—Africa. | LCSH: Feminism. | LCSH: Feminism—Africa. | LCSH: Sex role. | LCSH: Sex role—Africa.
Classification: LCC HQ755.8.F46 2020 | DDC 306.874096—dc23

Acknowledgements

I am grateful to the 28 mothers and fathers and their families who accepted my invitation to share their stories. Without their rich contributions, this book would not have been possible. I am also thankful to all the people who connected me with other key resource persons for this project to become a reality, my publisher and reviewers, and all the scholars who endorsed the book. My warmest thoughts go to you, my soulmate for your constant presence, and to you my daughter: you two are my bedrock! You have been an inexhaustible source and resource of warmth, hope, perseverance, and faith throughout the project, which took almost three years.

I am also grateful to all the previous generations of feminist writers, activists, and scholars from Africa and beyond who inspired me to become the feminist I am today. To you, my mother, thanks for teaching me to dance through the rain. Jërëjëf!

Anta, my sister. I love you more than ever. I dedicate this book to you and to our little gems.
— Rama Salla Dieng

My deepest appreciation to the contributors of the collection for their steadfast commitment to the book and to our copy editor Jesse O'Reilly-Conlin and designer Michelle Pirovich, whose tireless and skilled labour brought the book to life. Thank you again to my Demeter family of motherhood researchers and writers for providing the safe and sustaining homeplace that makes possible my motherhood scholarship. And finally much love and thanks, as always, to Terry Conlin, my most avid supporter, toughest critic, closest friend, and my partner in life.
—Andrea O'Reilly

Contents

Acknowledgements
3

Introduction
Rama Salla Dieng
11

Part I
Feminist Mothering Journeys
45

Chapter 1
Mothering Malaika: Thoughts on Feminist Mothering
Cheryl Hendricks and Malaika Eyoh
47

Chapter 2
There Is No One Way to Be a Parent
Nana Darkoa Sekyiamah
55

Chapter 3
Intuitive Feminist Parenting
Jael Silliman
61

Chapter 4
Feminist Parenting: A Memoir in Motion
Gertrude Dzifa Torvikey
73

Chapter 5
Colouring Outside the Binary:
Challenging the Imposition of Gender Binaries on Toddlers
Neela Ghoshal
87

Chapter 6
Becoming an African Feminist Parent
Satang Nabaneh
99

Chapter 7
A Muslim Feminist Mother
Astou Ka
107

Chapter 8
Parenting across Cultures, Continents, and Generations
Kathryn Toure
113

Chapter 9
"A Young Woman's Voice Does Not Break, It Grows Firmer"
Rama Salla Dieng
123

Chapter 10
Feminist Parenting from the Lens of a Muslim Woman
Kula Fofana
149

Part II
Parenting Is Political:
Of Feminist Mothers' Struggles and Resistance
161

CONTENTS

Chapter 11
The Necessity of Rage and the Politics of Feminist Parenting
Masana Ndinga-Kanga
163

Chapter 12
Growing into Motherhood
Sadaf Khan
177

Chapter 13
Thinking and Practicing Parenting;
or How to Do Right by My Child ... and Me?
Elena Damma
189

Chapter 14
It Takes a Village, as Long as You Have One
OluTimehin Adegbeye
203

Chapter 15
Feminism, Mothering, and Choice
Angelica Sorel
213

Chapter 16
Feminist Parenting: No Rock, No Egg!
Toucouleur
229

Chapter 17
Liberating One's Self:
Healing and Helping Others Do the Same
Joanna Grace Farmer
237

Chapter 18
"Just Wait until They Go to School":
Autonomy, Identity, and Feminist Parenting in an
Imperfect Society
Danya Long
251

Chapter 19
Sidestepping the Patriarchy:
Creating in Our Children a Critical Feminist Consciousness
Sehin Teferra
265

Chapter 20
Mother of Two: Reflections on Love and Loss
Nikki Petersen
271

Chapter 21
From Dreams to Action:
Creating My Own Happily Ever After by
Choosing to Adopt as a Young, Single Woman
Astrid Rosemary Ndagano Haas
279

Chapter 22
Feminism and Ecology:
A Complicated, Questionable Equation?
Elisabeth
289

Chapter 23
Why I Have Decided Not to Parent
(and Why I Won't regret It)
Elizabeth Wright Veintimilla
301

CONTENTS

Part III
Contributions from African Feminist Fathers and Children
307

Chapter 24
What My Mom and My Daughter Taught Me
Cheikh "Keyti" Séne
309

Chapter 25
Feminists Opened My Eyes
Oliver Ngweno
317

Chapter 26
The Struggling Feminists
Ousmane Diop
321

Chapter 27
"Work Hard for Your Little Girl" and
Other Dilemmas of Feminist Tightrope Walkers
Alioune 'Papa'
327

Chapter 28
Lessons on Feminist Parenting from My Nonfeminist Mother
Françoise Kpeglo Moudouthe
331

Afterword
Andrea O'Reilly
335

Notes on Contributors
349

Introduction

Feminist Parenting: Perspectives from Africa and Beyond[1]

Rama Salla Dieng

"In my view, the work of women in Africa is located at the boundary where the academy meets what lies beyond it, a third space where the immediacy of lived experience gives form to theory, allows the simultaneous gesture of theorizing practice and practicing theory, and anticipates the mediation of policy, thereby disrupting the notion of the academy and activism as stable sites."
—Obioma Nnaemeka 377

"We are moving on at a time of crossings, of seeing each other at the colonial difference constructing a new subject of a new feminist geopolitics of knowing and loving."
—Maria Lugones 75

Why an Anthology on Feminist Parenting?

The thirty contributors from diverse backgrounds, walks of life, and countries gathered in this anthology share powerful responses to the above questions by narrating their experiences of some of the challenges, dilemmas, promises, and compromises of parenting with a feminist perspective. This volume is one of the first collections published with first-person essays from feminist academics, industrial professionals or policymakers, activists or students, as well as allies; these essays describe very touching, beautiful, and sometimes painful stories of what it means and, more importantly, what it costs to become a feminist parent. In doing so, we aim to reclaim parenting as a necessarily political terrain for subversion, radical transformation, and resistance to patriarchal oppression, sexism, and racism.

This anthology will no doubt enrich the current literature on feminist parenting, in which voices of women and men from the geographic ensemble often referred to as "the Global South"—Africa and its diaspora in particular—have been missing. Therefore, this anthology fills a gap in the literature, as its essays seek to theorize feminist mothering, fathering, and parenting practices from the daily lives and experiences of parents in Africa, its diaspora, Asia, South and North America, and Western Europe. The countries represented in this volume are Ghana, Ecuador, Senegal, Cameroon, Ethiopia, Pakistan, Cote d'Ivoire, South Africa, Liberia, India, the Gambia, Uganda, Nigeria, Kenya, Germany, the United States, the United Kingdom, and France.

By presenting viewpoints from such diverse perspectives, the aim of the book is to record first-person narratives on the meanings and practice of feminist parenting in different socioeconomic, cultural, and political contexts. This collection takes into consideration a wide range of feminist viewpoints, identities, and practices, including African, queer, Islamic, secular, ecological, radical, liberal, and global. The book also discusses the ways in which loss, trauma, sickness, healing, and distance influence the feminist parenting experience. Moreover, it also explores alternative ways of parenting, not only through birthing but also through adoption, fostering, or caring for significant others.

Any parent, parent-to-be, or carer will be if not interested then curious about our anthology on feminist parenting. In fact, most of the scholarship on the topic focuses on feminist mothering rather than feminist parenting (Rich; Ruddick; Gordon; Reddy; Acholonu; Horwitz; O'Reilly; Green; Adichie; Oyèwùmí; Comerford et al.) or feminist/progressive fathering (Neal; Mutua; Richter and Morell; Moniz and Smith). This collection aims to complement the growing literature on feminist parenting and questions implicit assumptions concerning gender in the feminist mothering literature; it proposes that the concept of parenting is not simply the sum of mothering and fathering.

INTRODUCTION

The main attraction of this book is that the majority of its authors adopt a deliberately non-Eurocentric lens to their feminist parenting praxis, which is influenced by their rich, multicultural, and diverse histories. Thus, one of the main preoccupations of this anthology is to explore and question mainstream theory and practice of feminist mothering and fathering by paying a close attention to cross-cultural differences, similarities, and subsequent possibilities of other-parenting beyond the hegemony of Western models. Some parents offer an intersectional approach and analyze the impact of class, race, age, gender, religion, and location on their feminist parenting practice.

The process leading to the publication of this book has been a formidable learning experience and has offered critical insights on politics and power in knowledge production in the context of an international feminist collaboration. The main objectives of the book—beyond exploring the specific meanings each author attaches to their becoming parents—is to understand the authors' own accounts of what feminism means to them. More specifically, this book seeks to understand what feminist parenting means to the authors as well as the challenges they face given their gender, sexual, religious, and cultural identities. Last but not least, the book wants to uncover what it means to be a feminist parent in both theory and practice. Initially, each participant was invited to submit a short chapter on feminist parenting. Then, the format changed to accommodate the authors' personal writing wishes. For one, the contributors were more interested in sharing their personal experience than writing a more academic chapter, hence the call for personal narratives. In addition, most authors contacted in the initial stages appreciated the insights writing about the practice and practicalities of feminist parenting would offer, particularly concerning how to do feminist parenting every day as well as what its costs socially, economically, emotionally, and psychologically speaking. Indeed, the project and the product are somehow between and betwixt what was initially envisioned. This is a good thing because it shows feminist methodologies and collaborations are interested in honouring what is dear to feminists, the values of reciprocity, respect, flexibility, experience, as well as the desire to not commit epistemic violence.

In the present anthology, we tell our parenting journeys through the use of the first person, which allows us to recount the many nuances and peculiarities of our journey to birthing not only our children but also ourselves as new parents. These personal narratives are transcribed oral narratives and are faithful to African traditions of storytelling; they seek to recognize the agency of the parents and children as well as their experiences as a valid and prime source of knowledge on parenting.

African, Global South, and Western Feminism(s): Theorizing as Boundary Work

> "It is certainly possible to be an African and feminist. The question is how one as an African feminist navigates the politics of decolonization while working on the feminist enterprise of a world free from patriarchy."
> —Msimang 5

The novelty of this anthology is its use of personal narratives as a powerful methodological tool to render the pluralism of feminist parenting experiences—including other-mothering and fostering—in a way that evades Western-centric modes of theorizing. Indeed, making theories and defining worlds should not be the privilege of a happy few who can define not only the humanity of others but also accept or reject some theories, ontologies, or epistemologies as valid or not. Feminist scholars have contributed to problematising dualisms such as 'private/public', 'personal/professional', 'production/reproduction', among others. Feminist political economists such as Jennings 1999 have shown that most of these dichotomies are based on a 'dualistic ontology' in Western philosophy, which from the Ancient Greeks to the Cartesian 'invention of modernism', often separates social phenomena into distinct and mutually exclusive categories (Dualisms: 142-153). Feminist social scientists have therefore pushed for bridging the gap between these often artificial dichotomies and for the acknowledgement of the difference that time and space make in the production of economies and societies. It is important to acknowledge that claims to knowledge are indeed claims to power and that building theory as boundary work between different disciplines—in this case social sciences and the humanities—cultures, and worldviews is replete with political and ethical considerations. As aptly noted by Obioma Nnaemeka, the underlying questions are that "of provenance (where is the theory coming from?); the question of subjectivity (who authorizes?); the question of positionality (which specific locations and standing [social, political, and intellectual] does it legitimize?)" ("Nego-Feminism" 362).

Before discussing the experiences of feminist parenting covered in this volume, it is fitting to start with some conceptual clarifications. How would one define African feminism(s)? In attempting to untangle these concepts, a deliberate effort will be made to reflect on the politics of gender and knowledge production, since delineating these concepts also requires a focus on the power dynamics at play. It is important to state at the outset that this effort to define such complex concepts that cut across several disciplines is broad and incomplete and does not fully embody the nuances of the literature. The definition of African or Global South feminism(s) depends on the delimitation of both terms. In this collection, "Africa" does not just refer to "Sub-Saharan Africa," which is a problematic and racist construction because it homogenizes the countries situated south of the Sahara desert and excludes the Maghreb countries. We deliberately use the word "Africa" to acknowledge the fifty-five countries—and their diaspora—officially recognized by the African Union to celebrate concomitantly the diversity and the similarities between these countries. The terms "Global South" and "Global North" are also problematic. Such blanket conceptualizations may seem ambiguous not only because some of the countries labelled as part of the Global South are, in fact, located north of the equator but also because they often conceal the socioeconomic differences between the various countries labelled as such. Yet we decided to use these concepts, as Global South countries share similar legacies and a common history of organizing to resist and destroy the structures of colonialism and coloniality.

For understanding the scholarly writings on African feminism, and indeed gender in Africa, it is important to understand the reengineering of gender under colonialism as well as the shift in Western feminists' representations of African women. Indeed, the shift from "woman-as-heroine" in the 1960s to "woman-as-victim" in the 1980s reveals the mainstream focus on the "status of women" (Cornwall).

African feminists have provided a vibrant counter-response and have actively contributed to transform these representations of African women, and indeed gender, in feminist scholarship and organizing internationally. A founding moment for the emergence of Global South feminists was the conference held at Wellesley College in 1975. The conference was an opportunity for feminists from Africa, Asia, and Latin America to express their disagreement vis-à-vis some of the intellectual positions and social attitudes of certain American and European feminists and articulate a criticism against the homogenization of women and the universalism of questions relating to gender, race, and social classes. It was at Wellesley that African participants—such as Molara Ogundipe-Leslie, Bolanle Awe, Marie Angelique Savane, Fatema Mernissi, Filomena Steady, Nawal El Sadaawi, Niara Sudarkasa, Dina Osman, among others—met and decided to create what would become the Association of African Women for Research and Development (AAWORD) to support training, research and advocacy by and for African women (Leslie 4; Mohanty et al. 317). The creation of AAWORD was finalized in 1977, following meetings in Zambia and Senegal.

In addition, the work of Chandra Mohanty has also been instrumental. In "Under Western Eyes" and *Third World Women and the Politics of Feminism*, Mohanty contests the stereotyping of women from the Global South in northern gender and feminist thought (Connell). Feminist scholars such as Amina Mama, Ayesha Imam, and Fatou Sow were also influential in theorizing gender in the social sciences in Africa; other scholars also discussed African sexualities (Tamale) and queer Africa (Ekine), with a focus on creating a platform to discuss feminism in Africa (e.g., the *Feminist Africa Journal*).

It is almost impossible to define what "African" or "Global South" feminism means, as there are as many (African) feminisms as there are African feminists. In this book, we use the term "feminisms" to acknowledge this pluralism and diversity. In addition, we seek to define our feminism on our own terms and do not seek to establish an identity through resistance. In doing so, we take a political as well as an ideological stance, which is a way of acknowledging, showing solidarity with, and placing ourselves in the long line of previous generations of women fighting back against the sexism and patriarchy that has been forcefully imposed on them. This political charge is well acknowledged by the Charter of Feminist Principles for African Feminists itself:

> By naming ourselves as Feminists we politicise the struggle for women's rights, we question the legitimacy of the structures that keep women subjugated, and we develop tools for transformatory analysis and action. We have multiple and varied identities as

African Feminists. We are African women, we live here in Africa and even when we live elsewhere, our focus is on the lives of African women on the continent. Our feminist identity is not qualified with 'Ifs', 'Buts', or 'Howevers'. We are Feminists. Full stop."

Whereas before African feminists resisted radical feminism's vehement rejection of motherhood, (Nnaemeka, "Mapping African Feminisms"), we contend that mothering is neither nonfeminist nor unfeminist but a fundamental political decision with great potential to transform society at large—in the same way that choosing not to mother is also political.

African and Global South feminists are also part of the worldwide movement against sexism and patriarchy, yet their feminism is also preoccupied with addressing the specific structural problems in their societies, countries, and regions; moreover, being a feminist means different things to each of them. These feminists reclaim their differences and convergences, and they acknowledge their specific priorities and struggles based on their diverse contexts and identities while promoting collective action as well as reclaiming sisterhood and the legacy of their feminist ancestors who blazed the trail before them. For Amina Mama, who refers to Patricia McFadden's definition of African feminism, it is "the political praxis that emanates from a very cogent analysis of political, economic and social conditions that shape African women's lives" (qtd. in Salo 59). In the introduction of the volume *Feminism Is: South Africans Speak Their Truth*, Jen Thorpe reminds us that "feminism is a contested space ... it is a label that does not meet everyone's expectations, but it is a welcome home for others" (7). The Charter of Feminist Principles for African Feminists also supports this claim:

> As Feminists who come from/work/live in Africa, we claim the right and the space to be Feminist and African. We recognize that we do not have a homogenous identity as feminists—we acknowledge and celebrate our diversities and our shared commitment to a transformatory agenda for African societies and African women in particular. This is what gives us our common feminist identity.

African feminism(s) and Global South feminisms do not start with colonialism, just as the history of African and Global South societies do not start with their encounter with others. They have also survived coloniality and are actively resisting it. The rich legacies of feminist ancestors—such as Njinga Bandi of seventeenth-century Angola, Yennega of fourteenth-century Burkina Faso, the Kahina of seventh-century Algeria, and Lingeer Ndate Yalla Mbooj of the nineteenth-century Waalo Kingdom in Senegal, who led in public life in precolonial times—have been acknowledged (UNESCO). Yet there are many herstories that have been erased if not omitted deliberately, and there are many other women who are not of royal blood who would today be qualified as feminists. Although there are claims that feminism is far from being elitist and that it is for everybody, there also has been a deliberate erasure of voices of generations of women from Africa, the Caribbean, India, and Latin America because they contest mainstream feminism; thus, their voices need to be heard too, and the specificities and nuances of their diverse struggles must be acknowledged.

Today, one characteristic that unites many if not all feminists from Africa and the Global South, especially in postcolonial literature, is denouncing the "coloniality of power"—the racial social classification of the world population under Western world power and capitalist modernism, which has survived colonialism (Quijano 171)—as well as the coloniality of knowledge, or what be regarded as knowledge or not. Using the plural "feminisms" is, therefore, an effort to move away from building myths of homogeneous African and Global South families especially with the construction "poor women and children." Within such discourses of African poverty, the impetus "to develop" and to "rise" again economically has been made with the direct refrain that they should be done "under Western eyes." This centrality of self-collectively organizing against coloniality is illustrated in some of the most important work by women in CODESRIA (the Council of Social Science Research in Africa), which was founded in 1973; AAWORD, which was created in 1977; and DAWN (the Development Alternative for Women in the New Era), which was created in 1984. In addition, there are a few black, African, and Global South scholars who have also subsequently called out what Maria Lugones has termed the "coloniality of gender," which entails both capitalist and racist-gender oppression.

For a few African and black feminists, gender is not the most important social aspect in many African societies (Sudarkasa; Nzegwu; Amadiume; Oyèwùmí). Sometimes, and in certain places, they claim that other issues, such as seniority (age), matter more. In *Family Matters*,

Nkiru Nzegwu, for instance, argues that there is little focus on the family in the social sciences branch of African studies as compared to politics, governance, and development, which is not the case for the humanities branch of African studies. She then argues that "gender subordination in Africa over the last 60 years ... can be traced to European Colonial policies and African men's views and constructions of family" (2). She insists that in Igbo society in West Africa, for example, the mainstream normative model of family and labour relations dominant in colonial and nationalistic social policies totally reengineered women's identity "as that of a wife, and produced a developmentalist discourse and a series of nationalist and post-colonial policies that supported a dependency status of wives" (Nzegwu, *Family Matters* 4). She then interrogates the validity of gender everywhere; "What if the category gender is absent in certain cultures? Would the feminist perspective still apply in studying families and societies (based on the utilization of gender as an analytic category of explanation, the focus on women's experiences, and the placing in full view of both the assumptions and beliefs on the same cognitive frame)?"(*Family Matters* 9). In the same vein, Oyeronke Oyèwùmí questions "the invention of women" with specific reference to the Yorùbá society, which are also similar to the questions raised by Ifi Amadiume in *Male Daughters, Female Husbands*. Their writings posit that gender is fluid and changing in a dual sex-system. According to Oyèwùmí, Yorùbás do not do gender, and she contests the claim that African women benefited from colonialism; instead, most of them lost their judiciary power and property rights to the new patriarchal structures created together by local elites and colonial administrators (*The Invention of Women*). Yet Oyèwùmí's book has many methodological flaws, such as the use of an approach strictly based on a selective use of language to illustrate her claims and her defense of her matriarchal society when it is, in fact, profoundly patriarchal (Bakare-Yusuf; Nzegwu, *Chasing Shadows*).

Attempts to promote and celebrate alternative feminisms rooted in African cultural realities echo similar transatlantic efforts, which can labelled Afrocentric feminism(s). Womanism, for instance, is a term that was coined by Alice Walker in *In Search of Our Mothers' Gardens: Womanist Prose* as a response to second-wave feminism and to give visibility to the experience of black women and other women of colour, whose work and contributions to feminism were rendered invisible in mainstream media and historical texts. Walker defines womanism as "A black feminist or feminist of colour ... who loves other women, sexually and/or asexually Appreciates and prefers women's culture... sometimes loves individual men, sexually and/or nonsexually. Committed to survival and survival of entire people, male or female.... Womanist is to feminism as purple is to lavender (xii)." Womanist theories have been further theorized in Africa by writers, such as Ogunyemi (1985) and Kolawole (1997). For Ogunyemi, African feminists' experiences needed to be rendered more visible; the term "black feminist" represented more the realities of African-American feminists. Kolawole's view is that womanism gives lesbianism a centrality that is not representative of, and is even "strange" to, the heterosexual-marriage model and the family-centred worldview that are prevalent in Africa.

Not all African feminists embraced womanism, however. "Stiwanism" and "motherism" are different variants of feminism promoted by African women (Omolara Oqundipe-Leslie; Acholonu). The first one involves a "social transformation including women of Africa," which is also inclusive of African men. As for "motherism," it places motherhood at the centre of African women's feminism and reclaims "vital items" that have been omitted in the womanist discourse, "such as the family, the child, nature, mothering and nurture" (Acholonuu 90). Yet motherism, by its excessive attempt at specifying what is truly African, is essentialist, homophobic, and not progressive.

It would be reductionist to understand feminisms from the Global South as just reactive or reactionary. To fully understand African feminisms, understanding the realities of African feminists should matter more than comparisons with non-African feminisms as well as concerns over what African feminisms are not and cannot become. Such demarcations from global feminisms are rooted in the need for African and Global South feminists to build on the indigenous while addressing issues that are specific to their various societies. Therefore, Nnaemeka's expression of "nego-feminism" seems particularly accurate, since its focus is on proactivity not reactiveness; it advances crucial social issues collectively to try and find a balance and compromises, a giving and taking (Nnaemeka, "Nego-Feminism: Theorizing, Practicing, and Pruning Africa's Way"). This line of thought is close to Pumla Dineo Gqola's suggestion that postcolonial black and African theories on feminism are seeking to define innovative ways to address their own issues rather than just defining themselves as what they are not. Such feminisms "are no longer just concerned with writing back—to white feminists, to colonialism, to patriarchy, to apartheid, etc.—but are about refashioning the world in exciting ways where the difference within is not a threat but a source of energy" ("Ufanele Uqavile" 11).

Since the early 2000s, diverse variants of feminisms have blossomed on the African continent and in the diaspora. For Mina Salami, three main strands have emerged in this time to complement postcolonial feminisms (i.e., radical, Afrocentric, and grassroots). These three stands are the following: i) liberal feminism, which focuses on individual choices and freedoms but fails to address the consequences of neoliberalism; ii) millennial or fourth-wave African feminism, which is represented by young women organizing across the continent, including marches, student protests, blogging and vlogging, as well as artivism; iii) Afropolitan[2]; and iv) Afro-futurist[3] feminisms, which are forward looking and propose a transnational approach to feminism that is inclusive of (if not sometimes led by) the African diaspora.

Feminism has gained momentum globally. And more and more, African feminists are being recognised for their work including Chimamanda Ngozi Adichie whose TED talk "We Should All Be Feminists" and short book *Dear Ijeawele* have had a worldwide resonance. Social media has also contributed to new online and offline platforms of creativity, dialogue, and activism on feminist issues, such as africanfeministforum.com, MSafropolitan.com, HOLAAfrica.com, adventuresfrom.com, to name only a few. Currently, the #MeToo movement—which started a decade ago with Tarana Burke, an American civil rights activist and a victim of sexual violence herself—has sparked a worldwide movement to break the silence around sexual violence and harassment as well as in Africa and the Global South, including in such spaces as churches (#ChurchMeToo), mosques (#MosquesMeToo), and in the international development sector.

This anthology fills a gap in the literature, and its main purpose is to address feminist parenting in Africa and its diaspora, in India, the Americas, and Europe. Where these diverse feminisms have dealt with the question of parenting in geographically and mostly culturally specific ways—through what has been themed "nurturing," "caring," "rearing," "fostering," "social reproduction," and "other-parenting," among others—this book seeks to reconceptualize feminist mothering, fathering, and parenting practices and their global and local connections from the centre and from the margins.

The book also explores the perspectives of feminists from the Global North, particularly those working in Africa, as well as Muslim African feminists and queer parents. The Muslim parents in this volume reflect on their never-ending journeys to finding a balance between living according to their religion and ideological beliefs and practicing feminist parenting according to their African cultural realities. Although Islamic feminism has been under the scrutiny mostly of the West for the supposed tensions it raises between the secular and the religious, scholars, such as Margot Badran, call for a critical appraisal of that viewpoint and for a more nuanced understanding of the relationship between the secular and the religious, especially with the emergence of a more holistic cultural feminism. Such a point of view epitomises the current middle ground in feminism, where the religious and the secular meet or collapse (Badran 54). Adopting a feminist approach on women's rights in Muslim societies can be a real challenge, especially in Africa, where religious fundamentalisms have gained momentum (Sow). For Ayesha Imam, one crucial step towards avoiding essentializing Islam or leaving it to homogenising discourses is to make a distinction between the often conflated categories of Islamic and Muslim feminisms. Whereas the first is based on the Qur'an and is often dogmatic, the second is subject to social inquiry as well as multiple interpretations from different Muslim communities interested in practicing their religion according to their current realities.[4]

By presenting perspectives from such diverse perspectives, this book aims to record first-person narratives on the meanings and practices of feminist parenting in different socioeconomic, cultural, and political contexts.

Surveying the Literature on Feminist Mothering and Fathering

While researching for this introduction, I was struck at how Western-centric the literature on feminist parenting was. For Oyèwùmí, it is hardly surprising that "there is very little feminist research on the continent that can tell us about endogenous constructions of motherhood, because our scholars take their funds, concepts, and cues from

Western feminist research" (215). As an avid reader of literary writings from Africa and its diaspora, I passionately read Nnaemeka's edited volume—*The Politics of (M)Othering: Womanhood, Identity and Resistance in African Literature*—which offers a fascinating gender analysis of some of the most important texts in African literature. Through such themes as voice, agency, subjectivity, and sisterhood, the authors of this volume offer interesting insights on the central role that storytelling occupies in the production of knowledge and the role that gender politics has in making this knowledge peripheral. In doing so, the contributors show us how dichotomic constructions around power and positionality fail to capture the diversities of roles and situations women occupy in African societies, a reality acknowledged by this book. Another contribution of the collection is its forceful argument that gender politics shape knowledge legitimation as well as knowledge articulation through the use of language that can serve the purposes of othering. Reading Nnaemeka's edited collection reminded me of my school readings as I knew for a fact that African literature was replete with female writers narrating experiences of what being women means through their characters. Buchi Emecheta, Mariama Ba, Bessie Head, Nawaal el Saadawi, Calixthe Beyala, Ama Ata Aidoo, Ananda Devi, Tsitsi Dangarembga, and Chimamanda Ngozi Adichie have all explored the issues pertaining to women issues, including motherhood. Of course, African writers have written about feminist parenting long before feminism's arrival, as states Ama Ata Aidoo: "African women were feminist long before feminism" (323). That only some of these women identified as feminists or simply as "African feminists with a small f" (Emecheta) is not surprising, especially as feminism was long wrongly labelled as "un-African" by its detractors. Therefore, the present anthology seeks to link back to how these feminist trailblazers opened up new possibilities for the current generation of feminists; it also seeks, though, to leave an archive for the generations of feminists to come, whether they wish to parent or not.

In *What Gender Is Motherhood?*, Oyèwùmí discusses motherhood through the Igbo concept of "Ìyá" and claims that Ìyá, or "mother," is not originally a gender category. Germane to Oyèwùmí concept of Ìyá is that of "matripotency," or the "supremacy of motherhood," which is central to understanding Yorùbá epistemologies and cosmogonies. Ìyá is at the centre of her seniority-based system, which is also matrifocal and dominated by mothers. In this setting, matripotency "describes the powers, spiritual and material, deriving from Ìyá's procreative role" (58). After the birth of a child, Ìyá's responsibilities to their children are of an emotional, a metaphysical and a practical nature, and the most important of these roles is to provide for their children's position in her marital family, especially in patrilocal settings. The matripotent principle is more relevant when considered in relation to Ìyá's birth children. What about families with nonbiological children or parents? If seniority is the organizing principle, are blood bonds less relevant? In the other chapters of the book, Oyèwùmí deplores the role of a group of scholars who she calls "gender dictators" for being vectors for the production and dissemination of a scholarly work that promotes masculinist ideologies and male dominance (117-150). She also provides an analysis of the genealogy of Yorùbá names and naming practices to dissect the changes they went through and the apparition of gendered names in the nineteenth century as reflecting major social transformation (151-69). Oyèwùmí's book is a great contribution to the current scholarship on the many forms and shapes mothering and, indeed, motherhood can take when culture serves as a source, a resource, as well as "the meeting point of giving and receiving" (Senghor 34).

Another key and more recent contribution to feminist mothering literature is Chimamanda Ngozi Adichie's *Dear Ijeawele*—a manifesto she first published on Facebook in 2016 as a response to a friend who asked her a question about how to raise feminist children. The fifteen-suggestion manifesto was then published as a book in 2017. In the premise of the manifesto, the Nigerian author's not-set-in-stone definition of feminism, which she claims is always contextual to her, is based on her two "Feminist Tools"; the first of which is that every individual should start with: "I matter equally. Full stop." The fifteen suggestions are articulated around the following key ideas: that no mother should be solely defined by their motherhood status and that women and mothers should provide their children a sense of identity. They should also teach them to question language, reject likability, love their bodies and hair, and to denounce cultural and social prescriptions premised on selective reference to biology. Chimamanda also highlights the significant role that others play in the parenting, not merely as helpers but as carers too. Last but not least, she stresses the importance of educating girls about sex, the importance to giving and taking in love, as well as the importance of raising their awareness about differences between people early in life. These themes are discussed extensively in our book. We also believe that work still needs to be done to ensure that important sites of socialization, such as schools and religious organizations, work to reinforce the efforts made by feminist parents at home.

In her brilliant and powerful chapter "A Mothering Feminist Life: A Celebration, Meditation, and Roll Call", Pumla Dineo Gqola argues that mothering is a site of contradictions and shares her feminist mothering journey. She also pays a vibrant tribute to her feminist friends, who allowed her to find her own voice in parenting ("A Mothering" 13-33). Gqola beautifully narrates her feminist mothering journey while celebrating feminist sisterhood and paying a tribute to her feminist friends: "I could not have made it this far (in motherhood) without these feminists who hold my hand, hold my heart, and help me think into and out of a situation" ("A Mothering" 32). She also reflects on the challenges of raising boys (as many contributors in this volume) and articulates how maintaining a life-balance through keeping an individual identity outside of motherhood is crucial. She cites her friend Xoliswa's words, which summarize the spirit of a feminist parenting praxis:

> My baby has a life, and will have a bigger life. I have a life. We are building our life together. She is not my life and I am not hers. I have a great life that I have worked quite hard to design just as it is. I have no intention of giving it up. It's a relationship of love and nurturing and guidance and responsibility, and yes, there will be sacrifice, as there should be. But I will not sacrifice myself to motherhood. It would be a horrible thing to do to myself, and an injustice to my child. ("A Mothering" 30)

The parents in this book believe that societal change starts at home but extends far beyond it: parenting is an eminently political act. Therefore, we emphasize the importance of space, time and location in feminist parenting *realities*. For Oyèwùmí, it is not everywhere that there is such an obvious difference between mothering as an experience and motherhood as an institution, a difference stressed by Adrienne Rich in her seminal *Of Women Born: Motherhood as Experience and Institution*. Where Oyèwùmí argues that most African communities recognise matripotency, and therefore African feminists do not need to re-invent the wheel; for Rich, motherhood constitutes a patriarchal institution in which men control women's bodies for reproduction purposes, mothering centres on women's experience and is potentially empowering for the mother who can become an "outlaw of the institution of motherhood." Furthermore, for feminist scholar Andrea O'Reilly, who has extensively written on the topic of feminist mothering, not only is mothering conflated with motherhood in certain locations, maternity is mainly regarded as a patriarchal construct (*Matricentric Feminism*). Therefore, mothering anchored in feminism should consciously be aimed at destroying patriarchal motherhood and actively engage in restoring a mother's power and freedoms. This is why Fiona Joy Green calls for a "matroreform"—"the conscious process of (re)claiming mothering power by establishing alternative rules and practicing customs different to those (previously) prescribed by others" (90). Hence, O'Reilly suggests that motherhood might be more important for mothers than gender, and, therefore, mothers need a feminism of their own; thus, she calls for a theory of feminist mothering from a "position of agency, authority, authenticity, autonomy and activism" (*Feminist Mothering* 11).

In this volume, we also discuss parenting from the lens of feminist fathers. We consider fathers to be more than just biological fathers and parents; some fathers are actively involved in providing care as well as financial and emotional support to their children. As for the role of fathers, we reject the language of "light parenting" or "assistance." Fathers in this volume are feminist parents: they are not just helping or supporting their partner in raising the child. We used the term "ally" for lack of a better term to designate feminist fathers or what Mark Anthony Neal calls "progressive fathers" in *New Black Man*. In the present volume, we also included parents who adopted a child, parents who had experiences of other-mothering, and stories of former foster children, such as Keyti in Part III of this volume. In *Child Fostering in West Africa*, Erdmute Alber et al. describe child forstering as "a social practice allowing or obliging children to move to a household other than that of their biological parent(s) to stay there for long periods of time" (5). Child fostering plays an important social role in many Africans social groups because of the belief that leaving one's children with others (whether with relatives or at a *daara*, which is a Qur'anic school for young boys) is good for the children, as it disciplines them better and strengthens their character whilst reinforcing "the bonds between dispersed kin" (5). As for other-mothering, it is a common practice in Africa, particularly in West Africa, and among African-American communities for women to rear and care for children and families who are not biologically related to them.

Another key book on feminist fathering is Ato Quayson's 2008 anthology exploring the relationships between African and diasporic *Fathers and Daughters*. These beautifully written stories of fathering and be(com)ing daughters constituted a great source of inspiration for me. In one chapter, Simon Gikandi shares the following thoughts on the relationship between fathers and daughters:

> Stories of fathers and daughters ... are weapons against the stigma that we African men are condemned to bear in our sojourns in the world of the other. We know what this stigma is because we live it—the unquestioned assumption, irrespective of our family traditions and communal backgrounds, irrespective of our relation with our mothers, sisters and daughters, that we are the last custodians of an unrelenting patriarchy.... And yet, we know, as do our mothers, sisters, and daughters, that our connections to the rules of matrilinearity run deep and that our daughters are the constant reminder of our ordinariness. (68-69)

African feminisms promote negotiation, compromise, and inclusion; men are also considered as essential allies. In Africa, their role in parenting is particularly crucial, as African feminists invite men as partners in social transformation, including (or starting) with the domestic sphere (Nnaemeka, "Mapping Africa Feminisms"). In the literature, men who identify as feminist fathers are called different names. Some of the works cited here use the term "radical" (Moniz), "progressive," or "feminist" (Morell). Tomas Moniz, an American father started a magazine called *Rad Dads* initially to share stories on fathering that would present views that are different from mainstream and male-stream patriarchal constructs, which focus on discipline and heteronormative masculinity. The zine has since evolved to include all other genders and to offer a platform from all other marginalized voices in the parenting world, including parents of colour as well as trans and queer parents. In 2011, the book was released as a manifesto for "all men with babes in arms" to share their narratives in order to dismiss the clichés about "bumbling inept fathers" (*Rad Families: A Celebration*).

Voices of fathers of colour are indeed absent in the mainstream literature on parenting. In 2006, Athena D. Mutua theorized about "progressive black masculinities" to contest mainstream definitions of masculinity among black men, which hurt black communities as a whole, including black men and women. He also proposes that black men are oppressed by gendered racism. He defines progressive black masculinities as follows: "The unique and innovative performances of the masculine self that, on the one hand, personally eschew and ethically and actively stand against social structures of domination. And on the other hand, they validate and empower black humanity, in all its variety, as part of the diverse and multicultural humanity of others in the global family" (4). Marc Anthony Neal, for another example, discusses what it means to be a black feminist man and a black feminist parent in his book *New Black Man*. In his chapter "Bringing Up Daddy: A Black Feminist Fatherhood?" he talks about the impact of his inability to procreate a child of his own based on his definition of his own masculinity as a black man; the impact of the legacy of his father's not being an involved father but a breadwinner on his visions of fatherhood and manhood; and the prospect of adoption on his conceptions of black manhood and the parenting roles of fathers. He perceives his role as a father to his adopted child, Misha Gabrielle, as more of a co-nurturer rather that the general perception of a father in his community as the one who gets a woman pregnant and becomes the head of the family. He acknowledges that fathering is a feminist issue and decides not to contribute to "nurturing a patriarchal world" by refusing to review R. Kelly's *Chocolate Factory* as this would make him not a criminal but a "critical accomplice" of the singer, who is accused of a number of sexual misconduct cases. These voices on feminist parenting represent perspectives from black men in North America, yet the voices of African fathers who clearly identify as feminists still remain largely missing.

The literature on masculinities in African countries does not escape the centrality of white heterosexual patriarchy erected as the hegemonic form masculinity par excellence (Connell). As illustrated by Kopano Ratele in postapartheid South Africa, this white hegemonic masculinity, to which dominant forms of black masculinity were subordinated is crucial to understanding how women's subordination to men has been constructed as legitimate and normal. Hegemonic masculinity when conceptualized as multilayered and constantly changing or as plural (hegemonic masculinities) becomes a powerful analytical tool. For Ratele, the value of feminism in this context lies in its potential to engender "emancipated masculinities" in South Africa, which entails working through emotions and socioeconomic experiences that entrap men in harmful gender practices. As Ratele explains, such progressive black masculinities deliberately create new self-definitions to explicitly promote anti-sexism, anti-patriarchy, anti-capitalism in their anti-racist struggles (18). A key question to be asked in relation to this concerns the implications of not only moving beyond hegemonic masculinities but also the impact of hegemonic femininities (Hamilton et. al) or femocracies (Mama) on societies at large and on feminist futures.

Not only does the present book critically analyses fostering and adoption from the point of view of children and parents, it also incidentally discusses the phenomenon of missing fathers—a reality in many societies in the Global South (Richter and Morrell). For South African scholar Robert Morrell, the absent father argument has two difficulties: evaluating the real impact of the biological father on the child on the one hand, and countering the use of the children-need-their-biological-father argument to limit women's autonomy, on the other (Morrell 18). In addition, a recent study has found that fatherhood contributed to the development of positive and valorized sense of self in young fathers in South Africa (Endersten and Boonzaier). Therefore, this current book also discusses how the transformative potential of fatherhood can be collectively promoted to contribute to the construction of progressive masculinities with fathers not only providing for and protecting children but also actively contributing to the care of their families and society at large.

Being and Becoming a Feminist Parent and Doing Feminist Parenting Together with Others

Based on the above debates in the current literature, it is important to ask the extent to which *being* a mother, a father, or a feminist parent is an action verb that may fully recognize the powers of mothers, fathers, and feminist parents in public life yet is also shaped by social, gender, and cultural norms to influence how one *becomes* a mother, a father, or a feminist parent. In turn, how one becomes a mother, a father, or a feminist parent also spatially and temporally shapes social and gender norms. However, we also argue against the idea that becoming a mother or a father is the only way to become a woman or a man.

In *Gender, Sexuality and Mothering in Africa,* editors Toyin Falola and Bessie House-Soremekun aim to critically discuss the social construction of mothering, marriage, and widowhood in African societies, both in the past and in the present, and to analyze the process of mothering in relationship to language and its important role in African cultures. The authors argue that motherhood is an important rite of passage in African societies and that male and female members within households have specific roles to play based on the existing sexual division of labour. They explain this in more detail:

> Within households, even if gender roles are complementary, men are regarded as the heads of households while a woman has relevance as a mother and wife. She keeps traditions and kinship alive by bearing children and socialising them. As a bearer of children, she acquires respect within the household; as bearers of male children, she acquires prestige and ensures the stability of her marriage and the continuity of kinship and its traditions. Culture affirms the power that is available to women. (xvii-xviii)

Although this conception is still pervasive—that is, considering women's social worth only through their becoming wives and mothers—a few African feminists, including in this book, have discussed and challenged what Falola and House-Soremekun say in their introduction above, especially this sexual division of labour and the fact that women are often presented as powerful in the private sphere when they become mothers and wives. Even in fiction, the main female character of Cheikh Hamidou Kane's *Ambiguous Adventure* named "La grande Royale" is the chief's sister and a senior unmarried woman; therefore, class, caste, and seniority also matter in determining one's subject position in society.

Feminist political economists in particular have problematized such concepts as "the family" and "the household" as well as the division between production and reproduction. They have theorized that households, whether linked or not by conjugal social contracts, are sites not only of the negotiation of power but also of tensions and conflicts. Households, or the family, are also sites that render invisible women's labour for the daily and generational reproduction of labour and capital in African and Global South social formations. Hence, feminists have pushed for the recognition of this unpaid labour in national statistical accounts using various tools, including time use surveys. In addition, according to Shirin Rai and Georgina Waylen, feminist political economists have made the following contributions to feminist theory: i) recognizing the gendered nature of economies and understanding that economic crises are also crises in social reproduction, finance, and production; ii) evaluating the distributional impact of economic policies on women's rights; iii) investigating global shifts in women's work and their localized outcomes; iv) rendering visible the unpaid care economy and its benefits for families and communities; and v) producing evidence on how policymakers are (not) addressing this sector (6).

One may ask why "feminist parenting" and not "feminist mothering" or "feminist fathering"? We thought the first one would be more fitting because parenting is not the sole responsibility of mothers and fathers but also of communities, especially in contexts where there is a strong sense of collective being, becoming, and doing together with others. In this volume, our definitions of "mother," "father," or "parent" go beyond biology: we consider that being and becoming a mother is more than the sum of a father and a mother; it is more than just delivering a baby after pregnancy. In my native Wolof language, for instance, parenting (*jurr*) is more than the process following pregnancy (*ëmb*) and delivery (*wësin*). "Parenting" is also called to educate (*yarr*), to take care (*topoto*), and to cuddle (*nax* or *teette*). Therefore, parents (*wëyjur*) are more than just the father and mother; they also include senior relatives, grandparents, sisters and brothers, aunts and uncles, as well as their namesake (who plays an important role in the child's education). Similarly, the family (*njaboot*) is not just a nuclear one; it also involves the extended family, including the patriline (*geño*) and the matriline (*meen*). The maximal matriliny or uterine descent (*Xeet*) is opposed to the extended patriliny or agnatic descent (*Askan*). This sense of community in Senegalese Wolof families is well defined by Abdoulaye Bara Diop and also echoes Ubuntu philosophies in Southern Africa: *I am because we are.* This sense of community, especially the fact that parenting is something that is done with others is also evident in the proverbial African maxim that "It takes a village to raise a child." Many parents in this book appreciate the advantages and richness of bringing the collective back into parenting as a way to repoliticize it. Yet in the present volume, some do talk about the tensions and compromises that may arise in how one does feminist parenting together with others, for instance, when a parent decides to raise their children in a feminist way or decides to adopt and raise a child alone and away from heteropatriarchal norms. Therefore, sharing the experiences and reflections of parents about their own parenting is central not only for further theorizing about the lived experiences of parents but also for creating communities of solidarity and practice. It is also helpful in remembering that there can never be a generalizing discourse on parenting that could be relevant for all times and places.

Our book discusses and complements the existing literature by conceiving parenting as a necessary two-way process that enriches both parties in a fluid and dynamic relationship and that provides more reciprocal avenues for parents and their children to create and recreate together. Most contributors in our book agree that the way we parent is shaped mostly by socialization, education, and other influences. Becoming a parent and practicing feminist parenting are two different things. To become a feminist parent is difficult. It is a constant struggle against the self and the outside world. It is a battle against habits, asymmetrical power relations, domination, and societal discourses around parenting. It is about unlearning and relearning while considering the needs of both the parents and children.

This present anthology asks the following questions. What if we, especially those in or from the Global South, considered the tensions and possibilities between the passage from being a mother or a father to becoming a feminist parent? What are the promises and compromises between becoming a parent and doing feminist parenting? Does heteropatriarchal social validation deny parents their agency and sense of identity and intrinsic sense of self-worth outside of mothering (for mothers), and within fathering (for fathers)?

The Organization of this Collection

The chapters in this book are organized as an open dialogue between different generations of feminist parents sharing their experiences in three broad and complementary sections, including an introduction and an afterword. Part I centres on feminist mothering journeys, and Part II concentrates on the political dimensions of parenting through discussions around struggles and resistance of feminist mothers. Part III focuses on male allies, including feminist fathers' and children's experiences. The last chapter is an afterword by Andrea O'Reilly on the trajectories and topographies of feminist mothering.

Part I: Feminist Mothering Journeys

The ten chapters in Part I shed light on the mothering experiences of feminist parents across the globe. Eight of those mothers are African parents living on the continent or in the diaspora. Mothers in this section have a retrospective and prospective outlook about their journey to feminist parenting and the choices they have consciously made, such as the type of delivery, the choice of the child's name, the parenting style, and decisions about if they would be the primary care provider or not. All of the parents made the conscious choice to become mothers.

In Chapter 1, Cheryl Hendricks, a South African mother, shares a brief reflection on the ways in which feminism has shaped her ideas and practice of mothering her daughter Malaika. She narrates how mothering reinforced her determination to be a pan-African feminist and the ways in which it also influenced the choices of Malaika. For them, feminist mothering is about resisting patriarchal norms of motherhood, transforming gendered power relations, and providing those whom we mother with sufficient exposure to, and understanding of, difference and equality so that they can construct their own ways of being in the world. Feminist mothering liberates both mother and child, and situates them as actors of social change.

In Chapter 2, Nana Darkoa Sekyiamah reflects on growing up being fearful about sex, the possibility of becoming pregnant, the pain of having a missed miscarriage, her experiences of IVF, and her continued journey to becoming a parent through adoption.

In Chapter 3, Indian-American mother Jael Silliman highlights the four principles guiding her parenting style: a firm belief that women's rights are essential to social wellbeing; the idea that the personal is political; a commitment to challenging racism, classism, and all other inequalities through an intersectional feminist approach; and an obligation to strive towards the advancement of all women and vulnerable groups through solidarity and collaboration.

Chapter 4 is an autobiographical account of feminist mother Gertrude Dzifa Torvikey's struggles in raising feminist children in Ghana, which is patriarchal but also has a history of strong women with assertive voices. Such patriarchal tensions are felt not only in the household but also in schools and other institutions. Although she feels her story is not complete, it highlights her lived experiences as a feminist parent in Ghana.

In Chapter 5, Neela Ghoshal reflects on raising her child in Nairobi, Kenya. She describes her growing awareness of all the ways adults try to impose rigid gender binaries on children from an early age and to restrict children's freedom to be themselves and to imagine realities outside these binaries. As her child explores his own gender identity, Ghoshal struggles with an endless series of compromises; she seeks to encourage her child's creative and fluid understanding of gender while realizing that being assigned a binary gender from birth already closes some doors. The chapter asks hard-hitting questions about whether we need gender markers at all and suggests how we might affirm the existence of transgender, nonbinary, and intersex people by deemphasizing gender, starting with how we educate our children.

Chapter 6 is Satang Nabaneh's personal reflection on raising a son as an African feminist Muslim mother. It tackles the complexities and challenges of parenting from a distance, since Satang, who is from the Gambia, lives separately from her son while pursuing her doctorate in South Africa.

In Chapter 7, Astou Ka, a Muslim and Senegalese-American feminist mother, narrates her upbringing in Senegal and the role culture and religion play in her feminism parenting life in the United States. Through alternative lenses, she questions the institution of marriage and the place of women in it.

In Chapter 8, Kathryn Toure explores feminist parenting across cultures and generations. She asks, "How do parents and grandparents facilitate feminist parenting? How does a couple bring together cultural traditions to affirm children and promote diversity and equity?" Toure engages her children in conversation about feminist parenting, and she invites the reader to reflect on the paradoxes involved in challenging stereotypes, discriminatory systems, and existing hierarchies of power.

In Chapter 9, I speak about how becoming a mother led me to reflect more systematically about choice, power, and agency and to question any practice that was premised on the assumption that "this is how we do things" rather than on a conscious decision from the child or the parent. Growing up in a family with five sisters—and parenting between and betwixt continents and navigating through many professional and personal spheres—opened my eyes to the urgency of repoliticizing parenting and reaching out to and building synergies with other parents in order to learn and strategize together.

In Chapter 10, Kula Fofana shares experiences from two generations of Muslim polygamous households and how those experiences, coupled with the social, political and economic nature of the country, affected her concept of feminist parenting; she intends not to degrade the institution of polygamy but to understand it. She argues that the opportunity to relearn and unlearn previously held concepts of "how to" can be liberating, but changing the behaviour of men (and women) in patriarchal societies is where the real revolution lies.

Part II: Parenting Is Political: Of Feminist Mothers' Struggles and Resistance

In Part II, thirteen mothers discuss how the praxis of feminist mothering in an eminently political act. These mothers engage in alternative ways or approaches to parenting from mainstream prescriptions, which often place women and children under men's responsibility and control. Parents in this section have had to make difficult choices and sometimes unthinkable compromises trying to find a balance in their parenting style that encourages their children's autonomy. They also share tips about how to practice feminist parenting without losing one's mind and reflect about the legacy they are leaving to their children, their dream feminist futures, as well as the legacy they received from their own parents. The political economy of care is also incidentally discussed; the central role of caregivers, domestic workers, and family support systems are also recognized as essential. Paid and unpaid reproductive work is at the heart of patriarchal capitalism and has been discussed extensively elsewhere (Elson; Razavi; Folbre).

The mothers in this section approach parenting as a way to resist domination of all sorts including different kinds of patriarchies (e.g., indigenous, foreign, religious, and cultural), femocracies (Mama), hegemonic masculinities (Connell), and femininities (Hamilton et al).

These parents also (re)negotiate and (re)define the terms of their mothering in order to prioritize their (and their children's) wellbeing by finding ways to challenge the oppressive nature of motherhood in certain social and cultural contexts.

In Chapter 11, Masana Ndinga-Kanga understands rage as a fundamental feminist expression in parenting black girls and explores how the personal is intimately political in the intersection of race, class, and gender in South Africa. Her chapter challenges the popular narratives of self-sacrifice and submission in parenting discourse and presents a unique and vibrant alternative—a practical way of living feminism out loud in ways that help the black mother and child in a political economy where they experience silencing and erasure.

Chapter 12, by Sadaf Khan from Pakistan, explores the crisis of identity that is triggered by motherhood. It is a personal essay exploring the internal conflict faced by a new mother, who struggles to make peace with the change of perspective that threatens her identity as a professional, independent woman.

In Chapter 13, Elena Damma writes about her difficult journey of becoming a parent to her daughter in the wake of abuse, self-doubt, and loneliness. She explains how having a child forced her to actualize her agency and free herself from societal as well as her own expectations in order to be able to be the feminist role model she wants to be for her daughter. She shares painful insights into her journey of failing and becoming, and provides practical tips for single parents and how to engage meaningfully with single parents.

In Chapter 14, OluTimehin Adegbeye shares a moving narrative told in beautiful prose about how her feminist parenting emerged both consciously and subconsciously from loss as well as from conflicting ideologies concerning the family. She also speaks about her struggle to retain a sense of autonomy and a sense of joy and community that reach beyond the hetero-patriarchal hold of raising a child. She also shares her aspirations for her child as well as powerful visions of finding new love.

In Chapter 15, Angelica Sorel sees primary caregiving as a reproductive choice that women who become mothers should be able to take up as feminist parents. She describes how she was raised with normative ideals of a mother as the main carer, but that letting go of these ideas enabled her to develop a different way of mothering—one that presented her with fewer feminist contradictions than the conventional mothering model.

INTRODUCTION

In Chapter 16, Toucouleur reflects upon and draws lessons from treasured legacies and stories that unravel how generational change occurs sometimes. She proposes in her reflection to break silences, to own a voice of consciousness, to challenge the status quo, and to set boys and girls as well as women and men free. Toucouleur's reflection shows how feminist storytelling can be a way to empower both parents and children to remove gender gaps and to push towards a better world for every human being.

In Chapter 17, Joanna Grace Farmer explores the factors that increase resiliency and the ability to keep moving forwards despite adversity. It is also a testimony of a triumphant journey over tragedy and the commitment to help others to do the same.

Chapter 18, by British mother Danya Long, examines the tensions between facilitating a feminist home life and navigating an often skeptical wider (British, multicultural, and working class) community. It explores questions of how we support children as they come up against pervasive and damaging gender stereotyping, and argues that quietly but insistently existing in a fashion that challenges those limitations is a necessary act of feminism. Danya, though, remains cognizant that this is merely one aspect of feminist parenting.

In Chapter 19, Sehin Teferra, a single mother of two and co-founder of an Ethiopian feminist network, discusses her journey to feminist parenting based on following the principles of self-love, deepening our expectations of children regardless of gender, and standing up for justice and equality in small and large ways. Sehin encapsulates the core value on the path to feminist parenting by adopting a phrase from Chimamanda Ngozi Adichie—"learning to matter equally."

In Chapter 20, Nikki Petersen explores her complex feelings surrounding motherhood and mourning that arose for her when she lost her baby five months into pregnancy. Her experience not only sheds light on the way our society addresses miscarriage and loss but also on how we could better approach these difficult issues through a feminist lens.

In Chapter 21, Astrid Rosemary Ndagano Haas is half-Ugandan, half-Austrian, and football-loving urban economist still working on her PhD. Her chapter tells a lovingly hopeful story about how the journey of feminist parenting necessarily begins with a feminist journey of self-reckoning and of reconciling oneself with their insecurities, fears, and doubts, and then translating them into desires and aspirations. In this case, her story is one of adoption.

Chapter 22 by Elisabeth looks at the difficult relationship between feminism and ecology in a Western European setting. Social norms concerning mainstream feminism and ecology are strong and do not always converge, which puts more pressure on parents. Revisiting her own parental trajectory, the author insists on the importance of free choice as a central element of feminist parenting.

Chapter 23 by Elizabeth Wright Veintimilla considers the perspective of somebody who has decided not to become a parent in a world that is constantly imposing motherhood on women. The author describes her reasons behind making this decision and the ways in which she is planning her future outside of motherhood.

Part III: Contributions from African Feminist Fathers and Children

Part III comprises five chapters. The first three are by first-time diasporic African fathers, who narrate their parenting experiences. The last two chapters are written from the perspectives of children: the first shares their experience of being raised by a Kenyan feminist single parent, and the second is about being raised by a nonfeminist Cameroonian mother.

In Chapter 24, Senegalese artist Cheikh "Keyti" Sène narrates his journey as a father with his ten-year-old daughter, whose birth has led him to reflect on the condition of his single mom, which he witnessed while growing up. Through detailing the hardships his mother experienced as a divorced woman with children in a conservative society as well as the daily struggles he himself is facing while raising his daughter with different standards, Keyti tells us how he is learning about gender inequalities and his commitment to be an ally and change the norms and narrative.

In Chapter 25, Oliver Ngweno, a young man from Kenya, reflects on his experience of being raised by a single feminist mother, which adds to the diversity of feminist perspectives on parenting.

In Chapter 26, Ousmane Diop tells his story of coming of age in Senegal and then immigrating to the United Kingdom to live with his British feminist wife. He describes his partner and himself as struggling feminists. He also shares some of the many questions that those expecting their first child have.

In Chapter 27, Alioune 'Papa' explains how he became a feminist ally after growing up in Senegal and travelling to France at a young age. His experience of being fostered in a multicultural household in France, while still holding strong relations with his biological family, inspired and nurtured his feminist fathering beliefs and practices.

In Chapter 28, Françoise Kpeglo Moudouthe explores how he came to terms with realizing that his mother did not identify as a feminist, even though she had been the source of his inspiration and his emerging feminist praxis.

The volume ends with an afterword from Andrea O'Reilly, who has published extensively on the topic of feminist mothering. In her afterword, O'Reilly reviews the main theories of feminist mothering and argues that it has had a Western bias. In addition, the main literature is mainly theoretical and lacks empirical insights on the practice of feminist parenting beyond the Western world, which not only limits policy formulation but also hinders the establishment of transnational pathways to rethink maternal empowerment and invest in its repoliticization for social change.

Endnotes

1. Thanks to my two reviewers Annette Joseph-Gabriel and Roohi Khanna.
2. "Afropolitan" is a fusion of the words "African" and "cosmopolitan"; it was coined in Taiye Selasi's 2005 "Bye-Bye Babar" to refer to the Africans of the diaspora (those of African descent born and living outside of Africa). In the feminist literature, it gained popularity with Minna Salami's pan-African feminist blog MsAfropolitan, "which connects feminism with contemporary culture from an Africa-centred perspective."
3. This term was coined by Mark Dery in 1994 to refer to a "speculative fiction that treats African-American themes and addresses African-American concerns in the context of 20th century technoculture—and more generally, African-American signification that appropriates images of technology and a prosthetically enhanced—might, for want of a better term, be called 'Afro-futurism.'" (180).
4. For a discussion on Christianity, see Horn; Bompani and Valois.

Works Cited

Acholonu, Catherine. *Motherism: The Afrocentric Alternative to Feminism.* Afa Publications. 1995.

Adichie, Chimamanda Ngozi. "We Should All Be Feminists." *TEDxEuston*, 2013. www.youtube.com/watch?v=hg3umXU_qWc. Accessed 8 Feb. 2020.

Adichie, Chimamanda Ngozi. *Dear Ijeawele, or a Feminist Manifesto in Fifteen Suggestions.* Knoph, 2016.

African Feminist Forum. "The Charter of Feminist Principles for African Feminists." *AWDF*, 2016, awdf.org/the-african-feminist-charter/. Accessed 8 Feb. 2020.

Aidoo, Ama Ata. "The African Woman Today." *Dissent*, Summer 1992, pp. 319-25.

Alber, Erdmute, et al. *Child Fostering in West Africa: New Perspectives on Theory and Practice.* Leiden. 2013.

Amadiume, Afi. *Male Daughters, Female Husbands: Gender and Sex in an African Society.* Zed Books, 1987.

Amadiume, Ifi. *Reinventing Africa: Matriarchy, Religion, Culture.* Zed Books. 1997.

AWDF. "Charter of Feminist Principles for African Feminists." *AWDF*, awdf.org/wp-content/uploads/AFF-Feminist-Charter-Digital-%C3%A2%C2%80%C2%93-English.pdf. Accessed 8 Feb. 2020.

Badran, Margot. "Locating Feminisms: The Collapse of Secular and Religious Discourses in the Mashriq." *Agenda*, vol. 16, no. 50, 2001, pp. 41-57.

Bakare-Yusuf, Bibi. "Yoruba's Don't Do Gender: A Critical Review of Oyeronke Oyewumi's *The Invention of Women: Making an African Sense of Western Gender Discourses.*" *African Gender Scholarship: Concepts, Methodologies and Paradigms*, edited by Signe Arnfred et al., Codesria, 2004, pp. 61-81.

Comerford, Lynn, Heather Jackson, and Kandee Kosior, eds. *Feminist Parenting.* Demeter Press, 2016.

Connell, Raewyn. "Rethinking Gender from the South." *Feminist Studies*, vol. 40, no. 3, 2014, pp. 518-39.

Cornwall, A., ed. *Readings in Gender in Africa.* Indiana University Press, 2005.

Dery, Mark. "Black to the Future: Interviews with Samuel Delany, Greg Tate, and Tricia Rose." *Flame Wars: The Discourse of Cyberculture*, edited by Mark Dery, Duke University Press, 1994, pp. 179-222.

Diop, Abdoulaye Bara. *La Famille Wolof: tradition et changement*. Editions Karthala, 1985.

Gqola, Pumla Dineo. "A Mothering Feminist Life: A Celebration, Meditation, and Roll Call." *FEMINISM IS... South Africans Speak Their Truth*, edited by Jen Thorpe, Kwela Books, 2018, pp. 13-33.

Gqola, Pumla Dineo. "Ufanele Uqavile: Blackwomen, Feminisms and Postcoloniality in Africa." *Agenda: Empowering Women for Gender Equity*, vol. 50, pp. 11-22.

Ekine, Sokari, ed. *Queer African Reader*. Pambazuka Press, 2013.

Elson, Diane. "Progress of the World's Women." UNIFEM Biennial Report, United Nations Development Fund for Women, 2000.

Emecheta, Buchi. "Feminism with a Small 'f'!" *Criticism and Ideology: Second African Writers' Conference*, edited by Kirsten Holst Petersen, Scandinavian Institute of African Studies, 1988, pp. 173-85.

Folbre, Nancy. "Who Cares? A Feminist Critique of the Care Economy." Rosa Luxemburg Stiftung, 2014.

Gikandi, Simon. "A Voyage Round My Daughter." *Fathers and Daughters: An Anthology of Exploration*, edited by Ato Quayson, Ayebia Clarke, 2008.

Gordon, Tuula. *Feminist Mothers*. New York University Press, 1990.

Green, Fiona Joy. *Practicing Feminist Mothering*. Arbeiter Ring Publishing, 2011.

Hamilton, L.T., et al. "Hegemonic Femininities and Intersectional Domination." *Sociological Theory*, vol. 37, no. 4, 2019, pp. 315-41.

Horn, Jessica. *Christian Fundamentalisms and Women's Rights in the African Context: Mapping the Terrain*. AWID, 2010.

Imam, Ayesha. *The Devil is in the Details at the Nexus of Development, Women's Rights, and Religious Fundamentalisms*. AWID 2016.

Imam, Ayesha. *The Muslim Religious Right* ("Fundamentalists") and Sexuality. WLUML, 1997.

Imam, Ayesha, Amina Mama, and Fatou Sow. *Engendering African Social Sciences*. CODESRIA. 1996.

Jennings, Ann L. Dualisms. In J. Peterson & M. Lewis (Eds.) *The Elgar companion to feminist economics* (1999).

Kane, Cheikh Hamidou. *Ambiguous Adventure*. Penguin, 2012.

Kolawole, Mary E. Modupe. *Womanism and African Consciousness*. New Jersey: African World Press, 1997.

Leslie, Molara Ogundipe. *Re-creating Ourselves: African Women & Critical Transformations*. Africa World Press, 1994.

Lugones, Maria. "The Coloniality of Gender." *The Palgrave Handbook of Gender and Development*, edited by Wendy Harcourt, pp. 13-33.

Mama, Amina. "Feminism or Femocracy? State Feminism and Democratisation in Nigeria." *Africa Development/Afrique Et Développement* vol. 20, no. 1, 1995, pp. 37-58.

McFadden, Patricia. *The Challenges and Prospects for the African Women's Movement in the 21st Century*. Women in Action, 1997.

Mina, Salam. "What Is African Feminism, Really?" *Afropolitan*, 6 Dec. 2017, www.msafropolitan.com/2017/12/what-is-african-feminism-actually.html. Accessed 8 Feb. 2020.

Mohanty, Chandra Talpade. "Under Western Eyes: Feminist Scholarship and Colonial Discourses." *Feminist Review*, vol. 30, no. 1, 1988, doi.org/10.1057/fr.1988.42. Accessed 24 Feb. 2020.

Mohanty, Chandra Talpade, et al. *Third World Women and the Politics of Feminism*. Indiana University Press, 1991.

Moniz, Tomas, eds. *Rad Families: A Celebration*. PM Press, 2016.

Moniz, Tomas, and Jeremy Adam Smith, eds. *Rad Dad: Dispatches from the Frontiers of Fatherhood*. PM Press/Microcosm Publishing 2011.

Morrell, Robert. "Fathers, Fatherhood and Masculinity in South Africa." *Baba: Men and Fatherhood in South Africa*, edited by Lisa Richter and Robert Morrell, HSRC Press, 2006, pp. 13-25.

Msimang, Sisonke. "African Feminisms II: Reflections on Politics Made Personal." *Agenda: Empowering Women for Gender Equity*, vol. 17, no. 54, 2002, pp. 3-15.

Mutua, Anthony, D. "Theorizing Progressive Black Masculinities." *Progressive Black Masculinities*, edited by Anthony Mutua, Routledge, 2006, pp. 2-59.

Neal, Mark Anthony. "Bringing Up Daddy: A Black Feminist Fatherhood." *African Americans Doing Feminism: Putting Theory into Everyday Practice*, edited by Aaronette M. White, Suny Press, 2010, pp. 31-50.

Neal, Mark Anthony. *New Black Man*. Routledge, 2006.

Nnaemeka, Obioma. "Nego-Feminism: Theorizing, Practicing, and Pruning Africa's Way." *Signs*, vol. 29, no. 2, pp. 357-85.

Nnaemeka, Obioma. "Mapping African Feminisms." *Sisterhood, Feminisms & Power: From Africa to the Diaspora*, edited by Obioma Nnaemeka, African World Press 2005.

Nnaemeka, Obioma, ed. *The Politics of (M)Othering: Womanhood, Identity and Resistance in African Literature Paperback*. Routledge, 1997.

Nzegwu, Nkiru. *Family Matters: Feminist Concepts in African Philosophy of Culture*. State University of New York Press, 2006.

Nzegwu, Nkiru. "Chasing Shadows: The Misplaced Search for Matriarchy." *Canadian Journal of African Studies / Revue Canadienne des Études Africaines*, vol. 32, no. 3, 1998, pp. 594-622.

Ogundipe-Leslie, Molara. "Stiwanism: Feminism in African Context." *African Literature: An Anthology of Criticism and Theory*, edited by Tejumola Olaniyan and Ato Quayson, Oxford, 2007, pp. 542-50.

Ogundipe-Leslie, Molara. *Recreating Ourselves*. Africa World Press, 1994.

Ogunyemi, Chikwenye Okonjo. "Womanism: The Dynamics of the Contemporary Black Female Novel in English." *Signs*, vol. 11, no. 1, 1985, pp. 63-80.

O'Reilly, Andrea. *Feminist Mothering*. SUNY Press. 2008.

O'Reilly, Andrea. *Matricentric Feminism: Theory, Activism, and Practice*. Demeter Press, 2016.

Oyèwùmí, Oyèrónké, *What Gender Is Motherhood: Changing Yorùbá Ideals of Power, Procreation, and Identity in the Age of Modernity*. Palgrave MacMillan, 2016.

Oyèwùmí, Oyèrónké. *The Invention of Woman: Making an African Sense of Western Gender Discourses*. University of Minnesota Press. 1997.

Quijano, Annibal. "Coloniality and Modernity/Rationality." *Cultural Studies*, vol. 21, no. 2-3, 2007, pp. 168-78.

Rai, Shirin, and Georgina Waylen. *New Frontiers of Feminist Political Economy*. Routledge, 2014.

Ratele, Kopano. *Liberating Masculinities.* HSRC Press, 2016.

Razavi, Shahra. "The Political and Social Economy of Care in a Development Context: Conceptual Issues, Research Questions and Policy Options." UNRISD, Gender and Development Programme Paper Number 3, June 2007.

Reddy, Maureen, et al., eds. *Mother Journeys: Feminists Write about Mothering.* Spinsters Ink. 1994.

Rich, Adrienne. *Of Woman Born: Motherhood as Experience and Institution.* Virago Press. 1977.

Richter, Lisa, and Robert Morrell, eds. *Baba: Men and Fatherhood in South Africa.* HSRC Press, 2006.

Ruddick, Sara. *Maternal Thinking: Toward a Politics of Peace.* Beacon Press. 1989.

Salo, Elaine. "Talking about Feminism in Africa (Interview with Amina Mama)." *Agenda,* vol. 16, no. 50, 2001, pp. 58-63.

Selasi, Taiye. "Bye-Bye Babar." Lip Magazine, Mar. 3, 2005, thelip.robertsharp.co.uk/?p=76. Accessed 23 Feb. 2020.

Senghor, L.S. *Liberté I: Négritude et Humanisme.* Seuil, 1964.

Sow, Fatou. *Penser les Femmes et l'Islam en Afrique: Une Approche Féministe.* Akina Mama Wa Afrika, 2005.

Sow, Fatou. *Genre et fondamentalismes/Gender and Fundamentalisms.* CODESRIA 2018.

Sudarkasa, Niara. "The Status of Women in Indigenous African Societies." *Feminist Studies,* vol. 12, no. 1, pp. 91-103.

Tamale, Sylvia, ed. *African Sexualities: A Reader.* Pambazuka Press, 2011.

Thorpe, Jen, ed. *FEMINISM IS: South Africans Speak Their Truth.* Kwela Books, 2018.

UNESCO. "Women in African History." *UNESCO,* 2019, en.unesco.org/womeninafrica/. Accessed 8 Feb. 2020.

Walker, Alice. *In Search of Our Mothers' Gardens: Womanist Prose.* Harcourt Brace Jovanovich Publishers, 1984.

Part I

Feminist Mothering Journeys

Chapter 1

Mothering Malaika: Thoughts on Feminist Mothering

Cheryl Hendricks and Malaika Eyoh

Introduction

When I was asked to write this chapter on my personal reflections of feminist mothering, I was unsure what I would focus on. It was not a topic that I had spent a considered amount of time thinking about. Although I consider myself a pan-African feminist, I wondered if I had even engaged in a practice one could call feminist mothering. I deliberated on whether the focus of the chapter should be about what I consider feminist mothering to be—and whether how I mothered was indeed a feminist undertaking—or how my daughter, Malaika, experienced my mothering. How did my pan-African feminism translate in the home? I asked my daughter to write a page on how she experienced my mothering, and we have, therefore, co-authored this chapter. At the end this chapter is a brief reflection on the ways in which feminism has shaped my ideas and practice of mothering, how mothering has reinforced my determination to be a pan-African feminist, and the ways in which my mothering has influenced the choices of Malaika. Feminist mothering is about resisting patriarchal norms of motherhood, transforming gendered power relations, and providing those whom we mother with sufficient exposure to, and understanding of, difference and equality so that they can construct their own ways of being in the world. Feminist mothering liberates both mother and child; it situates them as actors of social change.

Making a Conscious Choice to be a Mother

The journey to become a black woman academic in South Africa, before the ending of apartheid in 1994, was not an easy task. There were very few black women positioned as lecturers or senior lecturers at the time and certainly none that we knew as professors (currently only 2 per cent of the professors in South Africa are black women). In Cape Town, where I lived and worked, we were a relatively close knit group of black junior lecturers supporting each other while competing in a highly cutthroat individualistic academic environment—an environment ready for neither black women professors or for black intellectuals more generally. In the 1990s, through the Southern Africa Political Economy Series (SAPES), based in Zimbabwe, a few of us were able to engage with powerful African feminists, such as Patricia McFadden, Ruth Meena, and Rudo Gaidzanwa. We defined ourselves as feminists and fought to have feminism included in the curricula of our respective disciplines in our universities. As we progressed with and/or completed our degrees, many of us were of the age when decisions about having children were being made. I can still recall some of those conversations and the conscious choices we, for various reasons, made to either have or not have children. Becoming a mother through the act of giving birth (for there are other ways of becoming a mother and of mothering), or choosing not to, is therefore a conscious decision for feminists. Making a choice to become, and when to become, a mother is the first act of feminist mothering. Deciding whether or not to be a mother breaks with the patriarchal assumption that motherhood is a natural destiny for women, that a woman's place is in the home, and that her roles in society are primarily located in the spheres of reproduction and nurturing. The ability to exercise choice is also closely associated with the freedom to do so and with the security that this provides.

Although I was in my mid-thirties when I gave birth to Malaika, I had already pondered about having a child in my early twenties and had named my prospective child then already. Malaika is a Swahili name meaning "my angel." The name was made famous in a Swahili song written by the Tanzanian musician Adam Salim in 1945, and is sung by, among others, the South African musician Miriam Makeba in the 1970s. The choice of my daughter's name is itself a reflection of my early pan-African leanings.

Although motherhood was definitely in my realm of personal identification, I also knew that it would not be the only role that defined me. I was curious about the world and wanted to study and travel. I was passionate about resisting injustice in all its forms, and I wanted to make a meaningful contribution to the transformation of our societies. I believed I could do all those things—have a fulfilling career and also being a mother. However, to accomplish these goals, I was also cognizant of the fact that I would have to delay having a child until at least some of my goals were accomplished. By this time, I was already approaching the age when women begin to worry about their fertility and hear echoing phrases about biological clocks ticking.

At the time, I thought I had prepared myself sufficiently to make the decision to have a child. In hindsight, nothing really prepares one for the changes that accompany having a child. It is not merely the physical transformation of one's body or the sudden realization of how much time a baby can consume that is a shock. It is also the acute awareness that your child is completely dependent on you for its physical, emotional, and intellectual wellbeing and that you are now responsible for its survival.

After my PhD comprehensive exams at the University of South Carolina, I had delayed writing my thesis. However, once Malaika was born, I completed the thesis pretty quickly. I became constantly aware of time constraints and I realized that if the thesis were to reach completion, I would have to write it while Malaika was sleeping. We lived in Toronto, Canada, at the time, so there was little in the way of family support.

Soon after I graduated, I was awarded a one year postdoctoral fellowship in the United States, which meant I would be in the United States during the week and in Canada on the weekends. There was quite a bit of guilt about this arrangement, as it had me away from my daughter for substantial periods of time. When her father and I separated, this became a bone of contention because her father could now claim primary caregiving responsibility during the period of my fellowship. At the time, however, it was what I needed in order to progress in academe.

The choice between childrearing and career advancement is one that the majority of women have to navigate. For those who choose both, it often comes at an enormous personal expense. This was no different for me. It was then, too, that I made a conscious decision not to have another child.

After the postdoctoral fellowship, I decided to move back to South Africa. Again, I had to make a conscious choice between staying with Malaika in Toronto or going home to where I thought I could make a more meaningful contribution (since I was unable to take her home with me at the time due to a custody dispute). Although it was one of the hardest personal decisions I have had to make, I do not have any regrets about it. Malaika remained in Canada with her father while I went back to my previous position at the University of the Western Cape. Upon my return, I spent a lot of time trying to get her to join me. This experience, I think, also contributed towards my feminist mothering. It was important for me not to feel disempowered or confined because I was a mother and to engage the custody dispute from a position of strength, even if that meant being away from Malaika for a year.

We do not cease being mothers when we are away from our children. Our care takes on different forms. It is, however, important that we nurture ourselves first so that we can be the best mothers we are able to be. Being a mother should be a conscious feminist choice; how we chose to perform the role of motherhood should be, too.

Mothering Malaika

Malaika joined me in South Africa a year later. Although she saw her father, who lived in Toronto, on holidays and he has always been present in her life, the primary responsibility for her wellbeing was now mine. I, however, had friends, family, and a helper in South Africa who gave me the necessary support I needed. Without that support network, it would have been extremely difficult to pursue the career I now have, which went from academe to the NGO sector and back to academe as a professor of politics and international relations. My work entailed a fair amount of travel on the continent. It could only be undertaken if others assisted with the caregiving responsibilities of motherhood—cooking, cleaning, babysitting, and ensuring that children got to school on time. I was, therefore, never a conventional mother. My child complained all the time that I was not at parent-teacher meetings or there to pick her up from school—I was not a "soccer mom." I saw my role more in terms of inculcating values, norms, and discipline as well as earning enough money so that we could live a relatively secure lifestyle.

Malaika, therefore, did not grow up in a home where there was conventional parenting or a sexual division of labour. In her father's home, he did the cooking and cleaning, and in our home, I was not the person undertaking these tasks, which has also affected the ways in which she has interpreted these roles—she does not align them to a particular gender.

I am an independent woman who has been able to succeed in career spaces in which men dominate. Malaika has often had to listen to me talk about the difficulties of my work environment and has had to listen to me prepare to give various talks. It was important that she and other young women see that they can be anything they want to be and that it takes commitment and passion to be successful. It is also important for our children to understand that we work not for individual success but for the greater good, that we are part of a collective, that we confront challenges while speaking truth to power, and that we seek to create a more just and equitable world. Having a feminist consciousness is about having a social consciousness.

I did not sit Malaika down to teach her. There is no curriculum for this. Feminist mothering is not about instructing. It is about creating different experiences and exposing children to diverse sets of gender and social relations through engagement, conversation, literature, film, culture, and so forth. It is about creating an awareness about power relations and promoting the values of equality and dignity that should be present in all our relationships. Malaika was part of our dinner table discussions; she also watched documentaries and movies with me, and had access to my books. Through the people I interacted with, she was also exposed to a world where gender constructions were debunked and where people could freely express their sexuality.

There were no men in the house, and she went to an all-girls school, which gave her the added confidence she now has as a woman. She did not have to spend her formative years competing with boys at school and/or competing with girls for their attention.

She did however have to deal with the race issue. South Africa was and remains highly racialized and a rather inward-looking society. She often had to deal with racism at school and within the extended family. In as much as I wanted to shield her from those experiences, I also wanted to equip her to be able to have the consciousness and emotional security to be able to traverse those encounters. In order to do so, I had to expose her to a world beyond the narrow confines of South Africa and its identity constructions.

In my own development, redefining myself as a pan-African feminist and working towards the greater good of women across the continent was liberating. Such a transformation enabled me to situate myself in a larger collective of people who have had similar experiences and who have been agents of their own destiny. I wanted Malaika to discover this, too. Only time will tell how far this has resonated with her, but telling signs are already there. I have seen her struggle with her identity construction and emerge from that inner contestation as a self-aware black woman actively claiming and embracing her identity.

I was, therefore, not surprised that she was one of the first students at her school to want to wear her hair in its natural curl, which led to many others at the school following suit and to a protest by learners at the school who wanted to wear their hair naturally that received international attention. There is now a change in the policies of many schools in South Africa for how black children can wear their hair. During the organization of the protests, I saw her grab my Angela Davies books and read them. A year later, Fanon and Biko disappeared from my book shelf. She was, therefore, grappling with the intersectionality of race and gender in South Africa.

By the time she entered university, I knew that my work as a pan-African feminist mother was largely done and that she now had to go and explore the world further on her own. Feminist mothering, I would like to believe, endowed her with the necessary confidence to chart her own way in this world. I look at her and I am proud of who she has become. I cannot talk about school plays or sports trophies, but I can speak about motherhood that enables a daughter to have the kind of sense of justice and equity that we need more of in the world. These are the values and beliefs that have emerged from my years of pan-African feminist mothering.

Malaika's Narration of Her Experience

Within the past two years of my life as a university student, the issues of patriarchy, gender-based violence, race, cultural sensitivity, and many other crucial social issues have come to the forefront of my thought process. Every day, I learn more and more about how to navigate my way through the world as a young woman of colour. Every day, I learn more and more about what that means and how my identity both disadvantages me in wider society and how it nuances my human experiences. It is in these day-to-day moments of learning that the idea of feminist mothering becomes increasingly important to me.

My mother is by her own definition a Pan-African feminist. This identity is something that has framed her life in a multitude of ways: from the work spaces she inhabits, the books she reads, the music she listens to, and the social spaces she finds herself in. Growing up, there was nothing I could do but follow these same patterns of behaviour. Without much note at first, as her daughter, I have absorbed her teachings in such a way that being in her presence allowed her to teach me without her lecturing to me. In her lifetime, she has done feminist work both in and out of academic spaces. Hearing her think aloud made me, as a youth, grapple with issues concerning women's place in both academe and wider society, women's place in South Africa and Africa at large, as well as what it means to be a woman in the world. These are ideas that I find myself wrestling with more now, and, increasingly, I relate my present ideas to the notions my mother originally provided me.

Her library spans the entire back room of our home and includes Toni Morrison, Angela Davis, Buchi Emecheta and Mariama Ba. When in need of something to read before I went to bed or caught the train, I looked to her library. Thus, my mother has been an avenue to work I didn't know I was interested in until I found it.

When I sit in my gender and writing classes in university this year, I'm increasingly shocked at the reading list. The ones I find myself enjoying most I look into who the author is. Almost without fail this year, my favourite texts have been authored by women I personally know through my mother, such as Desiree Lewis, Elaine Salo, and others—women I know as aunts and family friends. I now learn from them not only in private spaces but also in academic settings.

In my own day-to-day life, the teachings of my mother have become increasingly present. When in conversation with friends around the issues that affect us on a daily basis (whether it be what we're learning on campus or the fact that we can't walk through the inner city without being catcalled), increasingly I hear my mother and the women with whom she surrounds herself in my speech. I find myself increasingly able to look at social situations for not only what they are but also in terms of how I would want a feminist, nonracialized and, increasingly, more equal society to look like. This is a worldview I can accredit, in large part, to having a mother who defines herself as feminist.

Conclusion

Mothering is a conscious choice for feminists. Feminist mothering enables children to have a deeper love and respect for themselves and others as well as a deeper understanding of how the world and social and gender relations are constructed. It also provides them with a sturdy scaffolding for their own self-realization. Feminist mothering empowers both mother and child (and all others in the family) to be who they aspire to be and to fulfill their life's purpose. Feminist mothering takes courage, as society will judge and criticize those who break the stereotypes of how a mother is supposed to behave. It is important for young feminist mothers to build personal relations with other feminists who are able to guide and support them through the very tough choices they will inevitably have to make. Feminist mothering is fundamentally about teaching the norms and values of equality and about actively working to change the power dynamic between men and women and girls and boys. Pan-Africanism is about unity, solidarity, and dignity. Together, these are transformative values. They have made a lasting impact on me, and I trust that they will inspire my daughter and many others to continue to strive for the kind of society in which we all can enjoy the freedom, dignity, and growth that have been so long fought for and by so many.

Chapter 2

There Is No One Way to Be a Parent

Nana Darkoa Sekyiamah

I've always known that I wanted to adopt a baby. It's just always made sense to me. There are so many babies in the world that need a parent. Why make a baby of your own when you can take care of one that is already out in the world? Despite knowing this, I have always had this fear—will I regret not having a biological child of my own? Years ago, I sat in a workshop learning how to create digital stories. One of the trainers shared her story: "Every time I make a digital story, I realize that my one regret is not having a child of my own." That stuck with me, and that's a fear that I took on.

I first got married when I was twenty-five years old. When the marriage began to fall apart, my then husband said to me, "at least let's have a baby together." I was very clear that I did not want to do that. I did not want to feel encumbered in any way or have ties to the family that I was separating from. I went into my thirties with a sense of freedom; I was single and free to be whoever I wanted to be. Doctors would intermittently ask me, "Are you not going to have a baby?" I asked myself that question, too. At times, I asked my lovers, "Do you want to have a baby with me?" They always answered no. They wanted the dream— a house, marriage, and then a baby to complete the package.... And then after years of being single, I settled into a relationship in my late thirties.

We're Going to Have a Baby!

I screamed this when two lines appeared on the pregnancy kit that I had peed on a few minutes earlier. My partner came running to the bathroom. "What is it?" he must have asked. I pointed to the piece of plastic that had just caused a seismic shift in our lives. We hadn't been actively trying to become pregnant, but for a while now, we hadn't tried very hard to prevent conception. Scrap that. We had been downright careless. Our contraceptive of choice had shifted from condoms to a casual practice of the pullout method. [Spoiler: this is not an effective way of preventing pregnancy, and outside of a monogamous relationship where both partners have previously been tested and cleared of any STDs, it is also downright risky.] We had spoken about what we would do if we became pregnant and concluded that we would continue with the pregnancy.

My partner, though relatively young, and ten years younger than me, was keen to start a family, and I felt as if I was finally at a stage in my life where having a child would not automatically have a negative impact on my personal life or career. I had grown up with the notion that sex was bad, sex before marriage was a cardinal sin, and sex automatically resulted in pregnancy. My earliest memory of anything resembling sex education was watching a popular series on Ghanaian TV called *Osofo Dadzie*. Pastor Dadzie, the protagonist of the show, often punched a heavy, moralistic (dare I say judgmental) message. A common narrative would be a fast, rebellious teenage girl disobeys her parents, has a boyfriend, and falls pregnant; her boyfriend then abandons her, and the girl's life is destroyed. She has no choice but to have the baby in shame without the sanctity of marriage or the support of her parents and her community. She becomes a disgrace to the family and drops out of school very heavily pregnant without any support system. She is miserable. The viewer is left to imagine that the rest of her life as well as the life of her child is ruined forever. Whenever I watched such programs with my mum, she would turn to me and say something along the lines of "You see, that is what happens to girls who play with boys."

That memory, intertwined with my real life observation of a school mate who dropped out of school to have a baby, left me with a lingering fear of pregnancy. A part of me has always felt that I would only become pregnant accidentally, and, perhaps, that is what my partner and I had been subconsciously trying do. My bestie, a medical doctor, disagreed with this idea: "You can't seriously be doing the pullout method and think you won't fall pregnant!" And so after the initial shock of seeing two lines on plastic, we decided that we needed to celebrate. Both of us knew so little about pregnancy that our idea of a celebration was to go to our favourite wine bar at the time and drink a toast to our baby that we subsequently named SB—a combination of the first letters of both our surnames. It was important to me that any child I bore would carry my surname. Yes, I know my name is my Dad's name and comes from the patrilineal side of my family, but I also claim my name as my own, and, politically, it has been important to me not to take on the name of my partner—to know that any child of mine would also carry on my family name.

A Missed Miscarriage

Did you know that one in four pregnancies result in a miscarriage? I have known that for a while, but I only got to know that viscerally when I went to the gynecologist for what was meant to be my twelve-week scan. Pregnancy had been rough on me, much tougher than I had expected. No, I hadn't been throwing up or been visibly sick but I had been tired. So tired. All of the time. And nauseous, continuously. The only thing that seemed to hold back the constant wave of nausea was snacking continuously. Even before I had fallen pregnant, I had already made up my mind that pregnancy was not an illness and so I carried on with my life like everything was normal.

Normal for me was a fulltime job working as a communications manager for a global feminist organization, running a fashion label with my sister, curating *Adventures from the Bedrooms of African Women*—a blog about sex and sexualities—and running a small consultancy practice. Add to that a fairly hectic social life including weekly Rotary meetings, regular catch up with friends, weekly visits to my family, and a slightly obsessive gym schedule. In the first few weeks of my pregnancy, I took my Mum on a holiday to Benin and subsequently travelled to Mexico and Canada for work meetings.

On the day that I flew from Montreal to London, I was nine weeks and six days pregnant. I noticed that I started to feel better soon after I arrived in London. I wasn't nauseous anymore, and the tiredness was starting to lift. My initial thinking was that everything I had heard about starting to feel better at the end of the first trimester was true. I had no idea that the reason I felt better was because SB was no longer there. There had been one sign—light traces of pink in my underwear. Google told me that it was spotting, which could be a sign of a miscarriage, or, indeed, it could be nothing. I had hoped for nothing. I was wrong. The stillness in the doctor's face spoke volumes before she did: "I'm sorry. There is no heartbeat."

I had what is known as a missed miscarriage. All the remains of tissue were still inside me. I was given two choices. I could either wait for everything to come out naturally, or I could opt for surgery. I chose the medical procedure. It was meant to be day surgery, and I was to be in and out within four hours or so. One of my closest friends accompanied me to the hospital and waited with me for as long as she was allowed to. I woke up to a nurse saying, "I'm sorry. There was an emergency. You lost a lot of blood. We're going to have to keep you in and give you a blood transfusion." Later that night I woke up restless, with 101 thoughts running around in my mind. I did what I always do when I need to think about an issue: I wrote about my experience of having a miscarriage, published it on my blog, and cross-posted that link on my personal Facebook page.

Bloggers thrive on engagement—comments, likes, and retweets—but I was completely unprepared to deal with all the responses to my blog post and the stories women shared about their own experiences of miscarriage. There were stories of women who had had four or more back-to-back miscarriages as well as women who had had seven miscarriages and several failed IVF attempts. My heart broke over and over again. I cried harder than I had ever cried before. I wept for myself and all those women who had lost pregnancies they wanted to keep. I wept for women who felt they had to have a baby to feel complete. I wept for women who were scared that they were growing too old and wouldn't be able to have babies.

Unwanted Advice

Sharing my experience of a miscarriage also brought a lot of unsolicited advice:

"I didn't know you were pregnant. I wouldn't have allowed you to travel by road to Benin."

"Next time you are pregnant, don't travel for the first three months."

I tried to respond to that one: "But the doctor said I could travel."

"No, you should definitely not have travelled. Particularly by plane."

There was even more advice.

"You should try again soon. Don't wait too long to get pregnant again. Try right now."

Everybody meant well. I knew that, but all the advice wasn't helpful. What's the point in telling me that perhaps if I had stayed at home, if I hadn't gotten on a plane, if, if, if ... I might still be pregnant. Perhaps that pregnancy was not meant to be. Perhaps it was as the doctor said, "Just bad luck."

A Dream Deferred?

And so my partner and I decided to try and make another baby. The process this time was very different. We made several conscious choices. The first and the most important ones were to undertake a preimplantation genetic diagnosis (PGD) and in vitro fertilization (IVF). Like a lot of African people, we are both sickle cell carriers. There is a one in three chance that any child conceived by two people with the sickle cell trait could have sickle cell anemia—a condition that leads to constant illness and results in significant bodily pain. Patients tend to have short life spans. That was not a chance I wanted to take. I have lost close family friends to the condition. I have watched aunties consumed with grief while they lost one child, and then the next. I have myself lost a close friend to sickle cell. I don't want a life of illness and pain for any child of mine, and even though my Mum always told me from childhood "make sure you don't marry a man who is a sickle cell carrier," I ended up in a relationship with someone who had the same genetic trait that I had.

The first cycle of IVF was unsuccessful. The process showed that I had low to normal ovarian reserves for my age, and the most pragmatic solution if I wanted a healthy baby would be to try again, but for this second attempt, use a donor egg. I debated the pros and cons of doing this. I said to myself, "I might as well adopt. I've always wanted to adopt any way," but then I also thought, "If I use a donor egg, at least the child will be biologically that of my partner." But then that relationship came to an end.

And so here I am in my fortieth year, childfree, and still on the journey to becoming a parent. I've learned and relearned a lot on this path. I remind myself that there is no one way to be a parent. A parent is someone who raises and cares for a child and who loves a younger more vulnerable being. The journey to becoming a parent can take one through many different paths. All of them are legitimate—whether you become a parent through having your own biological children, through adopting or fostering, or through the constant care you give to children in your community.

My Models for Feminist Parenting

I am lucky to have many models of feminist parenting: legendary Ghanaian writer Ama Ata Aidoo and her feminist daughter, Kinna Likimani; the late Efua Dorkenoo, acclaimed anti-FGM campaigner, and her DJ-cum-lecturer son Kobina Graham; and feminist activist Hakima Abbas and her daughter, Jamila Abbas. In all these parents, I see elements of what I would want to be as a feminist mother—a mother who loves her child unconditionally and sees them as a human being as well as a person already imbued with their own personality and spirit. I want my child to grow up in a world that's a far better place than it is right now and to play a part in creating that world they want to live in. I want my child to also be a feminist activist and to speak up against atrocities wherever they may occur. I want my child to see the universe as her oyster and to be whoever she wants to be—her best self. I want to be a guide to my daughter, a feminist example, someone she can feel proud of and inspired by as well as someone who lives true to her own feminist values. I want my daughter to be comfortable in her body. To love her body however it is. I want her to be free of the issues that I have always had about my own body—that I am overweight, my stomach is too big, or my arms are too flabby. I want to surround her with an environment that tells her she is enough just as she is, and that if she isn't a she, that's okay, too.

Chapter 3

Intuitive Feminist Parenting

Jael Silliman

I came from the feminist activist world, but only later (in the late 1990s) when I became a professor of women's studies did I study feminist theory. When my children were young (between the 1980s and the year 2000), I practiced an intuitive feminist parenting style predicated on four basic principles: a firm belief that women's rights are essential to social wellbeing; the personal is political; a commitment to challenging racism, classism, and all other inequalities (now called intersectional feminism); and an obligation to strive towards the advancement of all women and vulnerable groups through solidarity and collaboration.

I grew up in Calcutta, India, in the 1950s and 1960s in a Jewish home—more culturally Jewish than religious. My grandmother was a teacher as was my mother, both strong women. My granny, barely five feet off the ground, stood her ground and was financially independent after my grandfather died unexpectedly in his mid-fifties. My towering mother, five feet seven with a formidable presence, taught at the convent school I attended. She still commands attention. My obstreperous father could not beat her into submission, although he did try. Violence—emotional, verbal, and sometimes physical—occurred in my home. My mother resisted, hit back, talked back, and eventually left him, despite the economically vulnerable future she faced.

I attended an all girls' school. Although my role models were women, these powerful, smart women did not buck the patriarchal social system, which was deeply entrenched. Gender clearly delineated roles. The professions for women were circumscribed—they could be teachers, secretaries, nurses, and doctors. I remember being quite taken aback when a woman banker attended one of my father's business parties. Until that moment, all the bank executives I had met were male.

When I received a scholarship to attend Wellesley College in the United States in 1974, feminism as a movement and practice became my world. Although I carry multiple and shifting identities—Jewish, Indian, immigrant, and now American citizen—it is my feminist identity that has been most formative and constant. My transnational feminist networks and my women friends have been my sustenance, support structure, and safe harbour throughout my life.

In the 1970s, Wellesley was a predominantly white, rich girls' school. We foreign students stood out as distinct from the typical white-Anglo-Saxon-Protestant (WASP) student. I was very involved with the South Asian students on campus and around the Boston area. Many miles away from home, I learned about the tumultuous political struggles gripping India. Indira Gandhi, prime minister of India, imposed "the Emergency" in India from 1975 to 1977, suspending elections and curbing civil liberties. It made no difference that Indira Gandhi was a woman. A woman leader and a feminist leader were entirely discrete entities. A feminist leader embodies the values and aspirations of the women's movement, which seeks to empower all women and realize their rights in an effort to create a more just society. Indira Gandhi personified the strong woman leader, whose ruling style was patriarchal: to prove herself worthy she outmanned the men dominating the political system.

Socialist feminism appealed to me, which sought to improve women's lives and strive to ensure equality for all women, especially the many women who did not have the class privileges I enjoyed. Combining feminist and new left precepts, I addressed the cultural and economic sources of women's oppression. Without economic independence, women can never enjoy full equality; women's liberation can only be attained as part of a broader movement for social, economic, and political justice.

I also embraced global feminism, which recognizes and challenges class and race privileges within and between countries while articulating the inherent limitations of Western feminism to address the needs of Third World women. For feminism to be relevant in a Third World context, it has to address the legacy of colonialism that undergirds the when three-year-old Shikha chose and insisted on wearing pretty, frilly, and preferably pink dresses. The more flounce and bounce the dress had the more she desired it! She made it clear that she enjoyed her stuffed toys and dolls more than playing with her trains and cars. I respected her choices while letting her know that she had and could make other choices. I gently told her she did not have to follow the way her friends expressed their gender identity.

With her beautiful Indian complexion and her head of thick, black, and straight hair, Maya was so different from her more girlie big sister, who also had a fairer complexion. From the outset, Maya was a tomboy, as she enjoyed many of the activities ascribed to the male gender: she loved sports and tumbling, excelled in gym, hated wearing dresses, and rarely played with dolls. She loved her blue denims and t-shirts and was less interested in reading books. Same environment, different choices! It is important for children to express their choices in the way they wish to look and what they choose to play. What they wear and the styles they choose are their experiments with self-representation.

The ways in which my girls represent themselves has shifted with time. As a late teen and a young woman, Maya dresses in a more sensual and overtly female manner than Shikha does. Shikha has given up the flounces and "dress drama" for a far simpler look. Nonetheless, I have tried to hold space for them to explore their own gender expression. Of course, against the backdrop of societally prescribed gender norms and pressures, this has not always been easy for them—but it has been their own journey, separate from mine.

From my girls, I learned that each child is unique and both nature and nurture make an individual. Some girls are more feminine, as are some boys, and some present the gender with which they resonate that may be different from their sex. Simply putting children into female and masculine slots does not work. It limits their sense of self and perpetuates patriarchy.

Skin Colour

Despite critiques of the dominant economic, social, and cultural paradigms that are upheld by many institutions, including the media, we live in its shadow. For example, dominant social norms reinforced by the media make it challenging for everyone, and especially children, to resist these subtle and not so subtle messages. As a parent, I have had to negotiate skin colour and brand image. Conformity as to ideals of beauty, body size, and appropriate dress is reproduced and policed in school and in broader society, where children are judged if they are too dark, too fat, and do not wear appropriate clothes.

We moved from New York to Iowa City, a progressive university town in the Midwest. Iowa City was very white. We stood out. Maya, who came to Iowa City at the age of two, was incredibly aware of our difference and began to feel the impact of being a darker child. A process of feeling lesser and different from became her reality. Although I did not grasp it until more recently, it was why she did not like me wearing Indian clothes, objected to my nose ring, and thought our house had too many voluptuous bare-breasted sculptures and paintings. Her friends poked fun at the many *Shaivite* and *Tantric* images, some of which were sexually explicit.

As a young brown girl surrounded by white peers, Maya started to question and internalize what it meant to be beautiful. In the third grade, she came home and suggested we dye her skin white. The honey-brown complexion that she was so proud of months before had suddenly become her deepest insecurity. In those moments I held Maya and reminded her of how beautiful she was. With daily reminders and affirmations of her own beauty, I tried to neutralize the messages she was receiving outside our home. Yet her skin colour was an ongoing insecurity for Maya in her younger years.

Shikha and Maya attended a summer camp, where Shikha was a camp leader. A girl who was to share Maya's tepee went to Shikha (not knowing she was Maya's sister) to complain about being put in a tepee "with blacks and browns." Shikha not only let her know that Maya was her sister, albeit of a different complexion, but that this racist attitude would not be tolerated. Shikha reported the incident and made sure that antiracism work was undertaken at the camp. A tear-faced Maya felt vindicated. I applauded Shikha for speaking up and taking the opportunity to go beyond the specific incident to address issues of racism at the camp. I assured Maya that although she had been the target of racism, this incident would help other girls like her to not meet the same discrimination, and if they did, they would feel more confident to report it.

When Maya was thirteen we moved to East Harlem in New York City. Her vision of beauty shifted again as she was immersed in a world with many brown and black people. Maya now prides herself on her honey complexion and reminds me of how influential my affirmations of her brown skin were on her as a young child. She is deeply involved in antiracism work and teaches primarily African-American children in New York City.

Brand Items

I had many arguments with my children when they wanted me to buy brand items for them. I tried to persuade them not to be free advertising for a brand. I suggested that designers should pay them to sport their logos. I told them that branded clothes made them look like everyone else. Finally, I told them that if we succumbed to buying these overpriced items, poorer kids would feel left out. Although I was able to make our shopping at Goodwill an anticipated and fun-filled shopping spree, I did not entirely win the brand battle with my preteen and teenager. I often succumbed to defeat. I could not win every battle—the girls had to win some too! Fortunately, my now grown-up girls do not sport brands, and when they receive them as hand-me-downs, they cut off the labels. Short-term losses lead to long-term victories.

Intersectionalities: Gender, Class, and Race

As an Indian (read brown) immigrant to America, I wanted my girls to grow up confident and to achieve the dreams and ambitions they cherished. I wanted them to be proud of their Jewish and Indian Hindu heritage (my ex-husband from India was an atheist but a Hindu by birth). I believed they could embrace their various identities and be richer for doing so. Diversity was integral to our lives, and I made a point to celebrate it. My home was filled with art from India, and we often ate Indian food. We celebrated some Jewish festivals, such as Passover. We went home to India regularly, where my in-laws celebrated Hindu festivals and performed a ritual *puja* (devotional prayer and offering) every morning in the *puja* room, which was dedicated to a multitude of gods and saints. We had friends from many countries and cultures. I tried to make my home a welcoming one and encouraged my children to have a cross-section of friends.

As I was engaged in feminist organizing and politics, my girls accompanied me on marches and protests and sat through numerous political meetings I attended. One day, after participating in several marches challenging restrictions on women's reproductive choices, I saw four-year-old Shikha marching around the garden shouting, "Not the church. Not the state. Women will decide their weight!" I had to explain to her that the march we had attended was for women to decide their fate. We had marched to demand that women could choose how many children they wanted to bear without anyone interfering with their choices. Thirty years later, the female body remains a contested site.

Around the same time period in the late 1980s, sitting around our Passover service, I asked, as is the Jewish custom of the children, "Who lead the Jews out of Egypt?" and Shikha proudly declared it was Martin Luther King! Although she was off by a few thousand years, she had grasped that the struggle for freedom was ongoing. I drew analogies between these struggles against tyranny. Although the Passover story is about an ancient period and King's struggle for racial justice was a more contemporary one, it remains vital to engage and show solidarity with those on the side of expanding freedom and rights and challenging injustices. This is a profoundly Jewish value, which has been celebrated and performed over the millennia during the festival of Passover; it commemorates the flight from slavery to freedom. Passover and having a *Seder* meal is a tradition I cherish and share with friends and family.

Sexual Diversity and Sex Education

I wanted my girls to be free from the inhibitions and shame around sexuality that was part of my teen environment in India. I dreamed that they would be comfortable in their own bodies and express their sexuality confidently. We had to struggle around fat shaming, in which bodies that do not conform to unrealistic notions of shape and size are ridiculed. Body shape and size were a source of struggle for Shikha in her preteen years as well as in her twenties. As I, too, have always struggled with my weight, I probably subconsciously compounded this problem.

Although I understand the feminist critique of body image as a way of undermining their self-confidence, I have not internalized this critique. I still struggle with my body not conforming to standards of body shape and size. My struggle with my own weight makes me more aware of other people's weight. My girls, while validating me, always check my thinking in this area.

I tried to make my children express their sexuality without any sense of guilt or shame. We discussed the negativity and unacceptable social policing of slut shaming, whereby women and girls are criticized if they are perceived to violate expectations of behaviour, expression, and appearance related to their sexuality. Often when I saw Maya wear what I would consider a very revealing neckline or a dress so short it looked like a shirt, I learned to hold back my opinion and/or judgment and not suggest she was dressing provocatively. The way I perceived her dress and self-expression was clearly a function of my own repression and social conditioning. I did share my insights regarding social attitudes and workplace realities related to dress. The ways in which girls and young women dress can be read and often misread, which makes them vulnerable to sexual abuse.

I spoke frankly with my children about sexual relationships and birth control. I believed that a precondition for a sexual relationship was for it to be protected, noncoercive, and mutually respectful. Growing up in America in predominantly university communities, I soon found out there was little I could teach my girls in this area. They had sex education in school and experimented with their sexuality from their middle teens with confidence.

By the time my children were growing up, the gay rights movement, which started in my college years, had made considerable social and cultural strides. Same-sex couples were a part of our everyday lives, and my children grew up not questioning this fundamental freedom. There are religious scriptures in Judaism that consider "homosexual sex" as an abomination, but I did not have to counter such beliefs because our household was not a religious one. When I visited Shikha in college, she introduced me to her friend Georgiana. The next time we met them, they were being referred to as George. When I rather naively asked Shikha if she did not find this shifting of gender confusing, she turned to me rather quizzically and said the following: "What is so confusing, Ma? You are smarter than that! When they are dressed as a boy we call them George. When presenting as a girl, they prefer to be called Georgiana!" Another lesson learned.

Despite the increasing social acceptance of gay rights, it was not till 2015 that the United States Supreme Court struck down all state bans on same-sex marriage, legalizing it in all fifty states. The transgender movement is in a much more nascent state; it promotes transgender rights and works to end discrimination and violence directed against the transgender community. Today, Maya reminds me of the importance of using pronouns correctly—they/them/theirs—and being more thoughtful of how we socialize gender expression.

Demonstrating Feminism Resilience and Strength

My now ex-husband began having a clandestine affair with one of my department colleagues and asked for a no-fault divorce. As I was under the mistaken impression that ours had been a loving and solid marriage of twenty-three years, I was first shocked and later devastated by his dishonesty and betrayal. Shikha had just left for college, and Maya was eleven. I left my tenured job so I could earn enough to obtain custody of Maya. Legally, we were both good parents, but in a custody battle, his drawing a higher salary than I did give him an advantage. Thus, I moved to New York City to be a program officer for women's rights and health at the Ford Foundation, where I earned a far larger salary than as an associate professor of women's studies at the University of Iowa. This job made the salary differential between us negligible, securing my right to Maya's custody. I could only imagine how devastating it must be for a woman faced with infidelity to also lose custody of her children because her partner earns more. This injustice is even greater when a woman has given up her economic independence, job, or career to do the heavy work of running the household and carework, which is also undervalued and unpaid.

My children were pretty distressed by the family upheaval. I had to show them that I was strong and independent and could carve out a new life for myself and attend to their material and emotional needs. Moving to New York City as a single parent was at first daunting, but with the help of a network of friends, it turned out to be much easier than I had anticipated. My mother, who lived with us in Iowa, also moved with me to New York City. This gave me more mobility than most single parents enjoy. By creating a new life for myself, I showed my children that when a woman is equipped to support herself and her family (a privilege too few women enjoy), she need not fear living as a single parent. They also learned the value of friendship and solidarity, which I had nurtured in my personal and political practice—it was sisterhood in action. Finally, the ability to work and invest in my passion—advancing women's rights—demonstrated to my children the importance of loving the work one does. My passion for my work provided balance and the base to build a new life when my past personal life had capsized.

My daughters have witnessed the many benefits I have derived from flying solo. They see that I live life on my own terms while I support them to build their own careers and networks of loving support. My children tell me the way I rebuilt my life in my late forties gives them greater confidence in setting the terms for the kind of life they wish to lead. Both are building their careers—Maya as an educator and Shikha as a lawyer working on human rights issues. They are passionate about their work and conscious of the need to be economically independent in a world where there are no guarantees.

Conclusion

My intuitive feminist parenting style is built on the principles and values I have outlined. These fundamental values have enabled me to steer through and negotiate the challenges of being a parent. As a parent, in interacting with my children, I have learned and grown. Shikha and Maya keep me in informed with the social and political realities they confront. I admire their perspectives and the ways they negotiate our rapidly changing world.

As feminist parenting is not authoritarian, my parenting has evolved to become a supportive and loving partnership of equals. Today, my children have as much to teach me as I do them. I stand in awe of the women they have become. I cannot take credit for the people they have become, just as I cannot take credit for their achievements and the contributions they make on a daily basis towards creating a more socially just world. However, I want to believe that my intuitive feminist parenting played some role in their making.

Acknowledgments

I would like to thank Suneeta Dhar, Radhika Rajan, Mallika Dutt, and Kathryn Toure for their review of my paper and their comments. I am grateful to my daughter Maya Bhattacharjee for her insights and suggestions to strengthen this paper.

interlinked homes, which, in later years, I called my "triangular experience." The first part of this chapter entails situating myself in my matriarchal grandmother's house together with my sisters and transitioning to my stepmother's house as well as exploring my relationship with my polygynous father who lived in a different house from his wife and his mother. In the second part, I situate the upbringing of my children in a monogamous conjugal home with a husband who is mainly absent. I also discuss how significant others—such as domestic workers, school teachers, and relations—mediate the parenting model that I envision and which I have tried to enact in a patriarchal society. In general, the lack of time has remained the main constraint for consolidating the gains I made in parenting my children in a manner that sets them apart from what society deems culturally normal. Moreover, the times I was away from my children also made them more independent in many ways.

Grandmother's Homestead

Today, I am a parent of three children—a son and two daughters. Although this in itself deserves a detailed discussion, it was my journey as a child and a dependent from five years old to eighteen years old that shaped my style of parenting today. I am not able to recall things that happened to me before I turned five. However, I do recall that it was at five that I was taken from my mother to join my father in Mepe, my hometown in the Volta Region of Ghana. Permit me to give a little detail of the story of my birth. My parents' marriage fell apart a few years after I was born. In fact, the breakdown could have been earlier. I got the details later. I was the reason the marriage broke down. I was born a girl.

My mother, together with her co-wife, had produced five daughters before my arrival. Three of these were my mother's children as she was the first wife. My father had had enough of the "girl nonsense." Sometime in 1979, my mother and her co-wife became pregnant approximately a week apart. In 1980, I was born. In the Eʋe tradition, barring any medical complications, a child is to be named on the seventh or the eighth day after birth by the child's father or male relation of the father, if the latter is not physically present. That was what my father was expected to do—give a name to a baby girl born on Friday. That was when the problem began. My father failed to call for the naming ceremony. He did not also give a name. His reason was that having had five other daughters, he had exhausted all the girl names he knew. Luckily for me, my mother's co-wife had a son ten days after I was born. So while my father was in his happy mood and preparing to name his first son, he asked my mother to bring me to be named. The marriage fell apart thereafter based on accusations of preferential treatment of the co-wife that my mother levelled against my father. My mother left the town with me to another part of the country. Five years later, my father demanded that I should be brought back to my hometown to attend school under his supervision.

I arrived at my grandmother's home. The house was full of my siblings and my uncle's children, all of whom were females. That household of about eight was female headed and female driven par excellence. Although I was raised in my grandmother's home, the place was only one of the sides of the triangular-shaped upbringing experience I had. My grandmother lived in a clan house, which also served as a point for traditional court hearings, and my grandmother took part in the proceedings. We the children served in the court as well, helping to serve alcohol after fines were imposed on offenders. We also sat in court to listen to the proceedings. I remember some of the proceedings resembled what I now come to know as a jury trial, but the children were not allowed to participate. Besides, only a selected few people sat in the enclosed place during the proceedings. I listened to these proceedings, many of which were domestic issues pertaining to child maintenance, divorce, abuse, and conjugal matters in general. Land matters were also adjudicated. I started forming my critical thinking from there on. I realized that although it was men who held the judicial powers in such cases, women from the clan, such as my grandmother, also contributed significantly to the proceedings. Offenders were often asked to bring assorted drinks including alcoholic and nonalcoholic ones as fines. The drinks would be served right there to the audience equitably and based on the individual's own capacity to drink. Children like me who sat throughout the hearings were not left out, although there was always a caution for moderation.

Apart from participating in traditional legal proceedings at an early stage, I also developed confidence and assertiveness through the types of games I participated in with my younger neighbours. One such game was football. I loved the game. I played football with boys who came to use our big compound for their activities, and my grandmother had no problem with it. As the youngest child at the time, my grandmother gave me few house chores, which gave me the space to play and express myself as a child.

Two religions also shaped my relationship with the cosmos and influenced me as a child and a parent, both of which took root from my grandmother's home. At the edge of the clan house where we lived was the clan's shrine. My grandmother participated in the shrine's activities. Sometimes, I followed her there. Whenever animals were sacrificed, my grandmother brought the meat home for cooking. Whenever the meat was cooked in the shrine, children were invited to take part in the eating. I realized I was beginning to learn to express myself in multiple ways, as I felt free taking part in traditional religious activities and also performing my duties as a child born to a Presbyterian father. I went to church regularly and also to the shrine when there was a performance there. I became more nuanced in reading the world, and this experience with two religions can be credited for this.

How does this affect my children today? It has been my principle that my children would only attach themselves formally to a religion when they turned eighteen and when they were adult enough to form their own opinions on religious matters and how they affect their lives. So apart from attending rite of passage ceremonies with them at church, I have not yet sent them to church. Although I was born into the Presbyterian Church and was committed to its ethos, I officially stopped attending in 2005 to allow me to reflect on religious messages that slap us in the face every day in our society. During that period, I found lies, the entrenchment of gender norms, fraud, as well as many other problematic things related to the practice of Christianity. I wanted to protect my children from religious dogmas because they could negatively influence their life and counter my efforts in raising them to grow into adults who appreciate the world in a more nuanced way. Nonetheless, they still received these same messages in school and through the media.

Residential Arrangements and Childrearing

Residential arrangements and household composition are critical in how a child is moulded. When I arrived in Mepe, I was sent to my grandmother's house where my other three siblings and my uncle's children also lived. My father's house was only about fifteen metres east of my grandmother's house, whereas my father's wife's house was located west of my grandmother's. My father played the role of the household head, and many things revolved around him. However, although my father provided financial support, both women—my grandmother and my father's wife—ran their households efficiently and were also in charge of disciplining the children under their care. It was only in a few instances when my father was called upon to punish a child. My father was a teacher; therefore, all issues to do with the education of the children were also his responsibility. In the evenings, we did our studies in my father's house, and he sat in the compound guiding the learning activities. I grew up having interaction in and being shaped by three households.

The fact that I lived my early days in a household where the women were autonomous in many ways, and where there was a semi-absent and semi-present father, helped me adapt later in life when I married a husband whose work took him to many destinations, both nationally and internationally. His work schedules led me to create a parenting style comprising of two people— a mother and sometimes a father.

I tried to keep my own children from internalizing the values of my patriarchal society. My parenting style is a mixture of many personal experiences. My father, a polygynous man, was patriarchal in all its dimensions. Although my birth was received as a misfortune as he wanted a boy badly, he still took my education seriously. However, when it came to major decisions about higher education, he clearly showed his biases. My personal history has elements of both empowerment and discrimination; therefore, I became more galvanised to institute gender awareness within myself first and then in others, including my own children. I would say, in general, that my resilience, resistance, assertiveness, and critical views have emerged because of my past experiences.

Parenting Other Children

For me, parenting did not begin in August 2011, when I had my son, but in 2002 when I completed a teacher training program and became a teacher. I became a breadwinner for about eleven household members at that point in time, which was due, in part, to rural-urban migration, as many of my siblings left the Volta Region to reside in Accra, the capital city. At that point, none of them had a meaningful employment. I was the only gainfully employed member of the household. Although I did not reside in the household, as I was teaching in another region, I had to send cash and noncash remittances to them. I had to visit the household on weekends to mediate and arbitrate several disputes that occurred in the household. The house itself was cosmopolitan in nature. In that house were my mother, my stepsiblings, my half-siblings, and my siblings. We had many frictions.

One of the key observations I made during my stay in my cosmopolitan household was the realization that some of the girls were competing among themselves over things I considered material—shoes, bags, makeup, and other beauty and fashion symbols. These were their key preoccupations rather than education and career enhancement. To change the thinking of the girls to more relevant goals, I instituted evening discussions about topics that brought the best out in them. I remember how I used to tell them "be a value added girl. Ask yourself what sets you apart from other girls."

Marriage: A Few Things Changed

I believe many people were shocked that I married. The journey of my next stage of parenting began after I became married, when key decisions are made. Before I completed studies at the university, I informed my course mates of my impending marriage, but many laughed it off. They never believed it. I realized that my views did not conform entirely to their views on marriage. In many discussions we had, they proclaimed me as a deviant. Such questions as whether a married young woman should use labour-saving technology—a washing machine— while her mother-in-law lives in the same house with her and her husband baffled me. When I said I would use it and would buy it with my own money, many thought that was too radical. They claimed that hand washing should be the preferred medium of washing, since the use of a washing machine would infuriate the mother-in-law. In many Ghanaian conjugal settings, mothers-in-law wield considerable power and could determine the success of the marriage; thus, they are revered and feared at the same time. It was from that level of the social construction of what marriage represents or should represent that I write my experiences as a parent, too.

Negotiating My Marriage Ceremony

Asserting my authority and arguing forcefully were not new things for me. When my then boyfriend threatened to leave me because I said I could only marry him when I completed university, I called his bluff. He was shocked. I was only three months shy of completing. I told him that if he could not wait for three more months after we had dated for six years, then we did not deserve each other. Subdued, he said he would wait. He did wait. Those were some of the early building blocks of my marriage and family life.

When my father gave my partner the list of items he needed to buy to initiate the traditional marriage process, I objected to the list. On the list were such items as lingerie and handkerchiefs, six pieces of Ghanaian wax prints, and other things. I thought the list was an insult to me and that my father was selling me, since I was a worker and had all those things and could buy many more for myself. Other items on the list appeared exploitative to my husband. I thought the amount of money my family demanded and the types of drinks he was to provide were exploitative. When I told my would-be husband I was revising the list, he said that providing the items was not a problem to him. I realized I was locked between two ends of patriarchy, with each calculating their own advantages of what my marriage would bring to them. I insisted and took out many irrelevant items while explaining to both my father and my partner why I needed to have a say in my own marriage.

A Son in August: It Takes a Village...

In the later part of 2010, I conceived. I was only three months into my master's program at the University of Ghana. It was tough—not only because I was a student but because I was bearing the experience alone, as my husband worked in another African country. When I did the test

I was still surrounded by several relations. The only significant addition was the presence of my husband in the household. My husband was raised single-handedly by very strong women—his mother, aunt, and cousin—at different periods of his life. He was trained to do house chores as women would normally do it. He cooks very well. He is very neat. He supports women's empowerment and condemns men who shirk responsibility towards their children, which he himself had experienced. He does not get in the way of my quest for higher education or advancement in any way. That said, I would state unequivocally that I have not engaged him more firmly on questions concerning feminism, partly because we did not stay together at the same space for a long time, as he worked outside the house or the country most of the time. His presence in the house anytime he returned from foreign trips revealed to me many things that I took for granted about coordinating childrearing and performing wifely duties at the same time. I think it was one of the most difficult times for the both of us.

As the weeks passed by, his complaints about the child crying and disturbing him stopped, and he took a more active role in helping out, especially at night. He would often take the baby, cuddle her, and play with her so that I could sleep. This he did willingly, as he observed the difficulties that I had to endure as a mother, a student, and a wife. By taking on some of the child-caring roles, which he was already very good at due to his upbringing, he has showed his commitment towards feminist parenting.

Giving birth to a girl also provided me with a new understanding of how gender constructions are applied to children while they are young. It was more pronounced for the girl than the boy, and I was on high alert to react to some of these subtle messages. For instance, some visitors to my house acknowledged the beauty of my baby girl but often said that she would become a Miss Ghana. Others suggested that her light skin would provide her with opportunities, whereas others implored me to braid or plait her hair. To these suggestions, I responded by resisting their attempts to make my daughter into an object to be ogled.

A Patriarchal School and a Feminist Parent

As a critical site of socialisation, the school has always been an area of concern for me. I realized that the school, which is also a space where religious expressions are transmitted, could undo the efforts I made at home raising my children. This is even more critical for me as my son started school at age one. Getting institutional care, I thought, was a balanced way of keeping my son safe while I used the rest of the time to pursue my schooling and look for work. In Ghana, the school and the church are inseparable, although on paper the country is supposed to be a secular one. So I pitched a camp at the local school to be sure that the energy that I put into rearing my child to become a balanced individual did not get neutralised in the school system. It was one of the most difficult things to do, since many of the things that happened in the school were more systemic than the individual teachers showing their gender biases in the way they interacted with children. From engaging teachers on how to discipline children to looking at their examination papers and checking their assignments, I seriously analyzed the school environment. Each issue presented a new opportunity to engage the teachers directly or, based on my assessment, to discuss the issue during a parent-teacher association meeting, a platform I used very well.

Usually, when my son returns from school, he would tell me the highlights of his school day. One day after he returned and got undressed, the following conversation ensued:

> Son: Mama, John [not real name] put his hands in Senam's [not her real name] pants, and my teacher beat John and Senam. John didn't cry, but Senam cried.
>
> I wanted to understand more.
>
> Me: Why did the teacher beat Senam?
>
> Son: I don't know.
>
> Me: It is sad. The teacher shouldn't have beaten them.

My son's description of the incidence horrified me, especially since the girl was also punished. I followed up the next day. I met the teacher. She narrated the incidence and added a more detailed dimension: Senam was reading aloud to the class. This was a kindergarten class with six-year-olds. The kids sat in pairs, and Senam and John sat together. While reading, Senam realized there was a hand in her underpants. She reacted, which attracted the teacher's attention. The teacher decided that punishing John and Senam was the best way to teach other kids not to engage in such acts. School kids in Ghana get corporal punishment, even though it is illegal per the rules and regulations of the Ghana Education Service. I was furious that the victim was punished and that the teacher saw nothing wrong with her actions. Yet I used the opportunity to educate the teacher on how her action would prevent other girls and boys from reporting abuse. I also educated her on victim blaming, which is the reason why only a little less than 5 per cent of sexual abuse cases in Ghana are prosecuted. In a subsequent conversation with my son, I explained to him how the incident between John and Senam should have been be dealt with.

School exercises and text books are good educational pieces to analyse how the school system reinforces gender norms. I have learned this not only as a student but also as a trained teacher. I have, therefore, made it a point to check those books regularly. I would provide my children counter-lessons. In teaching occupations, it is common to see a woman in a uniform for nurses and a man in a white uniform depicting a physician. While we discuss the professions together, I ask my son several questions, which he answers himself. One day, he told me, "Mama, my doctor is a woman. It means women can be doctors, too." In several practical ways, we arrive at a consensus. On one fateful day, he returned home with a homework assignment. The teacher wrote two sentences to be copied by the kids:

1. My mother cooks my meals
2. My father pays my school fees

To teach him resistance, I told him he should not do the exercise until I speak to his teacher. I also asked him the usual questions about the roles that have been assigned to a father and a mother in the sentences. He understood: "You mama, you pay my school fees too." I realized I was nurturing a feminist son. I became more determined to be more upfront and direct with my feminist childrearing.

My son often returns from school reminiscing and reenacting the activities that happened during the school day, which includes the singing of Ghana's national anthem and the recitation of the national pledge. On one of the days he recited the national pledge, I felt a sharp awakening concerning one of the lines in the patriotic piece. Ghana's national pledge was, of course, written by a man, and it goes as follows:

> I promise on my honour
> To be faithful and loyal to Ghana my motherland
> I pledge myself to the service of Ghana
> With all my strength and with all my heart
> I promise to hold in high esteem our heritage
> Won for us through the blood and toil of our fathers
> And I pledge myself in all things
> To uphold and defend the good name of Ghana
> So help me God.

The following lines shocked me. I had recited the national pledge since I was a child and know the lines in detail. But the politics behind the two lines never got to me until my son recited it:

> I promise to hold in high esteem our heritage
> Won for us through the blood and toil of our fathers.

For the first time, the lines of the pledge became a discussion point between my son and me. At the end of the discussion, we agreed that line should have read:

> I promise to hold in high esteem our heritage
> Won for us through the blood and toil of our fathers and mothers.

My son cherished the new version even better than the original version. I believe teaching him this will allow him to think more broadly about the contribution that each and everyone makes to the spaces they occupy—whether it is in the home or outside the home, for the family or for the nation.

Conclusion

My perspectives on bringing up well-balanced children happened in two specific contexts, one of which is very significant. I know my society is patriarchal. I experienced discrimination, gender-based violence, and other forms of oppression, some of which I concealed and others I resisted. These were innate in my character. However, living theory practically became a more revolutionary way of understanding and unpacking feminist thinking. The school helped a great deal. My children were conceived when I was a student, and I am still a student. Being a student gave me much impetus to question and critically examine actions and reactions on issues that relate to men and women. Although my own life trajectory has demonstrated some of the key issues feminists encourage women and girls to do—such as resisting, showing agency, questioning the status quo among others—doing these things provided me a "rebel" label in my family. However, it was not until 2010 when I took a course in gender did I begin reading feminist literature.

From there, many things followed. I credit my feminist approach to bringing up my children to this feminist literature as well as to my experiences in my many different households. My academic knowledge became part of my household, especially in raising my children. Parenting with a feminist frame will achieve success if it is aligned with antisexist childrearing approaches. These parents must critically examine what the school, the church, if they attend one, the media, and most importantly, family, friends, and neighbours who interact with their children teach them about gender norms. But, of course, it would be good if such feminist messages spread to them as well.

Chapter 5

Colouring Outside the Binary: Challenging the Imposition of Gender Binaries on Toddlers

Neela Ghoshal

Sometime around his second birthday, my firstborn child, precocious with language, made his first verbal effort to decipher gender. We were reading a picture book featuring cartoonish pictures of children. The kids on the page looked almost indistinguishable. They were grotesque caricatures of real children, with puffy cheeks, bulbous noses, and upward-tilted grins. One of them had long hair. "That is a girl," Chi announced, pointing to one of the kids.

Now that's a first, I thought. As a queer feminist mom, I had consciously taken some steps to deemphasize gender. When Chi was twenty months old and started preschool, I accompanied him for the first few days and observed while a teacher, reading to the children, pointed to pictures and asked questions. "What animal is this? A cat!" cried several children in unison. "And who is this petting the cat? Is it a boy or a girl?" "A girl," one child ventured, finger jabbing towards the isosceles trapezoid meant to represent a skirt on the illustration. "That's right!" exclaimed the teacher, pleased with her charges' increasing ability to identify and name things.

"But how are you sure it's a girl?" I asked myself inwardly. And what does it do to toddlers, whose brains we can manipulate like Playdoh, when we announce so definitively that a caricature wearing a trapezoid me to a better understanding of the multifold harms of gender fundamentalism, including the way we talk about "girls" and "boys" to our toddlers. Most people may fall into certain categories regarding their anatomy or their chromosomes, but a recognition of intersex lives demonstrates that boundaries are blurrier than we tend to think. And even when someone's anatomy fits into a box, there is no guarantee that their gender identity will agree to follow such constraints. So why the obsession, legally and socially, with the two boxes? Why the need to record the omnipresent F and M sex markers on our identity documents, our drivers' licenses, our children's school registration forms? Why the need to ask pregnant strangers "Is it a boy or a girl?" Doesn't this insistence on binaries hurt not only intersex people but also trans people and anyone whose gender presentation may not match the sex they were assigned at birth? Couldn't it, in fact, hurt everyone—even people who identify as heterosexual, cisgender, and endosex (nonintersex)—by boxing them in and presupposing their identities aren't in the least bit fluid and malleable?

A friend forwards an article describing how Ontario, a province in Canada has issued its first "nonbinary" birth certificate to an adult who rejected their male gender marker; my colleagues in the global LGBTI rights movement draft a new set of principles—the Yogyakarta Principles plus 10—recommending that governments stop including gender markers on birth certificates and identity documents altogether; and my mind races with a sense of possibility. That's where my head is: imagining a world beyond gender, for all of us, for all our children. We would not all have to disown a personal sense of gender in this ideal world, but binary sex or gender categorizations would not be inflicted on us at birth. Gender would be malleable, disconnected from sex, and probably more marginal to how we define ourselves or are defined by others.

That's where my head is, but my feet are nestled in the dry Kikuyu grass in my suburban Nairobi estate, where upwardly mobile Kenyan parents send warnings around on the neighborhood WhatsApp group about a Nickelodeon program featuring a gay character and then applaud the state censors for blocking the distribution of the program because it may harm our children. In Nairobi, the older children alight from yellow school buses in thoroughly gendered uniforms: skirts for the girls and trousers and ties for the boys. In Nairobi, my own marriage is marked by a more stereotypically gendered division of labour than I ever expected. My children see me (and female nannies) doing most of the childcare and the logistics and the day-to-day routine maintenance work of a family while my husband dips in as the fun roughhousing dad, dips out and then dips in again in that other classic male incarnation—the disciplinarian—before dipping out again. And, of course, it's not just Kenya that is conservative around sexuality and gender. Back home in my own country of birth, the Trump administration is busy forcing transgender women inmates into male federal prisons where they have a one in three chance of experiencing sexual assault (Tourjée); state government officials are exiling trans children from the school bathrooms in which they feel most safe and comfortable. Meanwhile, the American Urologist Association continues to rabidly defend medically unnecessary surgeries on intersex children. They chop off the offending bits of "oversized" clitorises to "normalize" babies and make them fit in to a society built around sex and gender binaries, despite protestations from intersex activists, such as Pidgeon Pagonis, who says in a compelling Human Rights Watch video testimony that "I can imagine that I would love to have my intersex body intact."

I make endless compromises with myself, with my adopted culture, and with the people in my life. My husband likes to remind me when I get too gender bendy for his comfort level that we had a conversation, shortly before getting pregnant, in which we rejected the idea of raising a child without a fixed gender. It's true: we did. I remember it well. We were on holiday in South Africa in 2013, drinking wine, of course, before dinner in Stellenbosch. I'd just read a news story about a Toronto couple that was refusing to publicly announce the sex of their child, Baby Storm, which seemed revolutionary. (This was before my queer friend in London and her partner decided to do the same.) They wanted to let the child decide for themselves (Green). "I admire that," I said, "but I'm not sure I'd be ready to deal with the judgment from others." "I see where they're coming from," agreed my husband, "but the problem is that they might cause their child to suffer through experimenting on it." This is the same argument that is made to convince the parents of intersex children not to allow their children to live with their bodies intact. A chorus of accusing voices rises up: who wants their child to be an experiment?

Our first child was born—a water birth in a Nairobi hospital—and before we knew if he had all his toes and fingers, of course, someone exclaimed, "It's a boy!" He received the male marker on his armband and in his documents. I never seriously considered any alternative. We chose first and middle names from our Indian and Kamba cultures, which offer few gender-neutral options—no Kennedy or Kyle or Storm for this Nairobi-based family.

With their gender markers and their names, I recognize I have already closed certain doors for Chi and his younger sibling, and they'll have to push with all their might to reopen them in the future, if they choose to do so. In my endless series of compromises, I try to avoid padlocking those doors. I haven't banished the notion of "girl" or "boy" from my vocabulary or my children's, but my politics demand that I approach them with nuance. I try to use the terms sparingly, a tough act when phrases like "good boy" rather than "good child" are virtually seared across the cerebral cortexes of English speakers. (This is not the case in Kikamba or Kiswahili— Bantu languages in which pronouns have no gender, and neutral terms like "child" and "person" have much greater currency, although Kenyan cultures have developed other ways of policing gender from early on.) So when Chi asserts that the long-haired, bulbous-nosed caricature is a girl, I reply cautiously, "Well, it's probably a girl, although it could be a boy."

A few months after first "recognizing" the girl caricature, Chi declares, "I want to have long hair, but it's for girls." "Boys can have long hair, too. Anyone can have long hair, sweetie," I reassure him, pulling up photos on my laptop of his cousin who lives on a hippie commune in Virginia—an eleven-year-old who with his ironic smile and streaming flaxen hair looks ready for a career in an indie-rock band. Cousin Zad is three-fourths white and bears little resemblance to my brown-skinned, curly haired child, so I also pull up images of black boys with dreads, including the wild luxurious curls on teen actor Jahking Guillory as well as the classic image of a pensive Bob Marley, whom Chi has so admired ever since his father started singing him "Three Little Birds" as a bedtime lullaby.

I stick to the usual gendered pronouns in describing my child, although he's not old enough to affirmatively agree to such pronouns, and a part of me regrets imposing them on him. But sometimes it is Chi who pushes the boundaries, who demands of me a radical openness regarding gender and fluidity.

At age two-and-a-half, Chi asks for a bike, so I hunt around on

Facebook marketplace groups for a used one. It turns out my friend Dana is selling her daughter's old bike for two thousand shillings, three times cheaper than anything else I can find, "if he doesn't mind purple," she qualifies. He certainly doesn't: I have been observing his preferences. One of his pairs of hand-me-down jeans was falling down around his slender hips, so we headed to Woolworths to buy his first belt. In the boys' section, the belts were dreadfully dull—nothing but plain brown or black, even for two-year-olds. Chi made a beeline to the girls' section, pointed out a pink, sparkly Barbie belt adorned with green and yellow hearts. "I want that one," he said with certainty. "Are you sure?" the cashier asked me. "That's a girl's belt." "We're sure," I said, slamming down my credit card on the counter, no further questions, Your Honour. So the purple bike, at the unbeatable price? No problem.

But then a few days later, in the car, Chi asks: "Mama, is me a girl?"

"Why do you ask?" I peer back through the rearview mirror.

"Bilal says I'm a girl."

Bilal is a neighborhood kid, a three-year-old who seems rough around the edges; he often runs around the estate unsupervised and wheels his bike up onto our curb, without training wheels already. Indeed, I've heard Bilal asking Chi why he's riding a girl's bike.

I ask, "What do you think? Are you a girl?" And Chi says firmly, "Yes."

"Well, you can be whatever you want to be," I tell him. I don't read too much into this. Between parents and school and a nanny and the estate, I have no idea who's giving Chi his information about what girls and boys are or what those categories even mean at this age. But I realize from his innocent questioning how easy it is to fit children into boxes and to force gender fundamentalism on them. Many parents, even progressive ones, may automatically respond, "Don't let Bilal bother you. Of course you're a boy."

And then he gets more creative. It starts with lollipops. He announces one day, "Lollipops are for girls." Where does this come from? He must have seen a girl eating a lollipop, but how he decided that was a particularly gendered food item, I have no idea. I tell him lollipops are for everyone, although it's not healthy to eat them frequently. It comes up again a few days later. He is still just past two-and-a-half. We are reading *The Little Engine That Could*, and one picture shows lollipops— "good things to eat for the little boys and girls on the other side of the mountain!"

He says, "When I am a girl, I will have a lollipop."

The response that comes out is "Okay. But even as a boy you can have a lollipop, just not very often."

"Lollipops are for girls and boys?" he asks with some incredulity.

"Yes, lollipops are for everyone." I imagine a candy-coloured, gender-bending world where you can just change genders and get a lollipop. Then maybe you change back and get a mandazi.

The questions and comments come more frequently between two-and-a-half and three. A few times, he asks, "Mama, am I a girl?" Then he says, "Mama, I want to be a girl." And although I passed on raising a nongendered child, I tell him "You can be a girl if you want." He wants to paint his nails, and I say yes. (When we go to the neighborhood shop and he picks out green nail polish, the shopkeeper asks him "Is that for your girlfriend or for you?" Right, because it makes so much more sense that a two-year-old would want nail polish for his girlfriend than for himself.)

He is clearly turning the issue of gender over and over in his developing brain. I sometimes wish I could get inside and see exactly what's going on. "I want long hair," he says. "When I'm big, I can have long hair like Nyambura," who is his best friend next door, a six-year-old cradle snatcher with long braids who wrote him his first love letter. (Dear Chi, I love you. Kiss kiss kiss, Nyambura.) "Sure, you can," I respond; when he's asked for dreadlocks like Bob Marley, I've told him he can only have them when he's older and can take care of his hair by himself.

Then he grabs the neckline of my long red and blue sundress. "When I will be a girl…" He pauses. "When I will be big, I can wear a dress." What just happened? Why the adjustment away from gender fluidity mid-sentence?

"Yes, you can, Chi. When you're big, you can wear a dress."

The dress thing, it keeps coming up. As he gets closer to three, he wants me to buy him a dress, and I evade the question. We do live in Nairobi, not Brooklyn, and I'm not sure how ready I am to push this close to the edge of "experimenting on your child!" But he presses me, plaintively: "Mama, why will you not buy me a dress?" I struggle with what I may be denying him. Is he gender nonconforming? Will he turn out to be transgender? Or is he just a three-year-old who is falling in love with the world and all that it has to offer, and is wondering why on earth some of those things—especially the beautiful, sparkly ones—should be off limits to him?

I just keep trying to blur the limits. When he asks, "Does Wambui have a penis?" I respond with nuance, "Well, probably not, because I think Wambui is a girl, and most girls don't have penises, but some do!"

"Do some boys turn into girls?" he asks openly. "Yes, some boys turn into girls. And some girls turn into boys. And some people don't want to be boys or girls!" I explain. And then, being three, he carries on according to his own irrepressible logic: "And some people turn into walls! And some trucks turn into trees!" "Mm," I mull it over, "I've never seen a person turn into a wall." (The next generation will find my living-thing fundamentalism hopelessly outdated.)

My husband, who believes in the basics of gender equality but is bewildered by my increasingly gender-radical brand of feminism, gets annoyed: "You're confusing him. He needs to understand that boys and girls are different. That's part of the world he lives in." The accusation gets worse in an argument: "You're brainwashing our son to think that boys and girls are the same." It begins to affect our marriage.

I try to explain that even if one finds gender categories useful, they are overused, and I just want our children to have options, to not be boxed in. The way we talk about gender—even, at times, among feminists—remains so rigid, at least in the corners of the world that I inhabit. My feminist lawyer friend in New York picks up her keys from the coffee table and says, "Let's get the boys ready and head to the library." Why "the boys" as such an unquestioned marker, when we don't use other characteristics in the same way? She'd never say, "Let's get my Jewish children ready." Although race is far from irrelevant in our societies, kindergarten teachers do not call out "blacks and whites, line up for lunch!" What if we classified our children by their belly button types? For example, I run into a colleague at the supermarket with my kids: "This is my innie, and my outie is over there in the milk aisle," I tell them. "I have three kids, two righties and a lefty."

Gender didn't have to be the fundamental dividing line in society. The Nigerian anthropologist Oyèrónké Oyěwùmí argues that in precolonial Yorùbá society, "gender was not an organizing principle.... Rather, the primary principle of social organization was seniority, defined by relative age." Third-person pronouns in Yorùbá do not indicate sex; rather, different pronouns are used to "make a distinction between old-

Oyěwùmí, Oyèrónké. *The Invention of Women: Making an African Sense of Western Gender Discourses*, Minneapolis: University of Minnesota Press, 1997.

The Yogyakarta Principles plus 10. Nov. 2017, yogyakartaprinciples.org/wp-content/uploads/2017/11/A5_yogyakartaWEB-2.pdf. Accessed 10 Aug. 2018.

Tourjée, Diana. "Trump's Prison Guidance Puts Trans Inmates at Greater Risk of Abuse," *Broadly. Vice*, May 14, 2018, broadly.vice.com/en_us/article/8xeax3/trumps-prison-guidance-puts-trans-inmates-at-greater-risk-of-abuse. Accessed 10 Aug. 2018.

Chapter 6

Becoming an African Feminist Mother

Satang Nabaneh

I became a feminist because I believe in the equality among men and women and everyone in between. However, as a result of the continued marginalization and exclusion of mainstream feminism, my feminism is *African*, which pays attention to the interaction between age, sex, socioeconomic status, rural-urban divide, as well as other factors. African feminism (a boiling pot of diverse discourses) is concerned with the African situation. Intersectionality is critical as a starting point to account for how the patriarchal nature of African societies serves as a barrier to women's full realization of their potential.

As a girl growing up in the Gambia, I realized from an early age that girls and boys as well as women and men were not treated the same. I find myself, like the majority of African women, in spaces where I continuously have to contend with gender challenges, stereotypes, prejudices, and discrimination. Girls are taught to grow up to become so-called good wives and good mothers, which form important constructs of a woman's identity. Such socialization is deeply reflective of entrenched traditional attitudes and perceptions about the role of women in society, which I had to continually challenge. I am privileged that my parents taught me early on not to be afraid of speaking up.

Thus, my understanding of feminism deeply influences how I raise a son in a way that reflects, represents, and respects the values espoused by feminism. I currently mother my son, Mahy, mainly from a distance due to pursuing a doctoral degree in the United States (US), where I currently live with my husband. This idea of distance mothering ruptures the very foundation of the ideal Gambian family, which is premised on the notion that good mothers must physically remain with their children. How then does my feminism and all that it has to offer interact with sociocultural norms of the role of the mother?

In this chapter, I try to address this question by examining my parenting journey. A reenactment of the concept of motherhood that allows the pursuance of educational or economic goals necessitates the sharing of childrearing responsibilities with others. And this chapter interrogates and critically reflects upon the challenges arising out of my location as a black graduate student and Muslim mother to a son living in another country.

Self-identifying as an African Feminist Mother

Often when two adults meet in the Gambia, the first thing they ask each other is "how are the children?" This method of greeting is also similar in most parts of Africa. I am an African woman. I am from the Gambia; it is mainland Africa's smallest country, a snake-shaped West African nation tucked literally inside of Senegal with just a tiny coastline touching the Atlantic. The Gambia is a deeply patriarchal society that perpetuates the dominance of the alpha male as the protector and the provider. A woman's identity is structured around that of her husband; it is also defined by what religion and the society expects her to be and do.

I then moved to the U.S. where I gave birth and partially raised my son, Mahy. My husband later joined us as well. Coming from a deeply religious country and living in a very liberal environment in the U.S. at a young age and becoming a student mom have had deep implications on how I view parenting. Both my husband and I are from Muslim backgrounds; we teach our son about Islam but try not to reinforce patriarchal tendencies and actions.

My husband would not label himself as a feminist but as a traditional African man and Muslim dad. His decision does not necessarily have implications on my feminist position and the desire to raise our son as a feminist, as we have definitely tried to set up our marriage and household as an equal partnership. To us, that means balancing our family life by dividing tasks and what needs to be done. Although we do not have jobs that pay the same amount, each of us is able to bring whatever we can to the table. But it is important that our son sees both parents handling money, paying for groceries, or settling the restaurant bill. We want our son to learn that money is earned by both parents through hard work. This is particularly important to me, as I grew up in a household where my father had a white-collar job and my mother stayed at home. Although my mother handled the money, she was equally able to make her own money through petty trading. She became the breadwinner of the family for a while when my dad lost his job and was able to take care of her four children. This experience taught me the value of respecting and supporting each other for contributions that each can make, and I hope our son learns this valuable lesson as well.

Upon discovering I was expecting, I was not particularly concerned about the sex of my child. I promised myself that whatever the sex was, I would raise my child to believe in herself or himself, to value hard work and dignity, and to refuse to be defined by society's good man or good woman standards. The moment I looked into my newborn son's eyes, I knew that his future rested on what we did from that moment on—how we brought him up, what examples we would set before him, and what values we would inculcate in him. The question for me from then on was how I nurture my son in such a way that does not reproduce and rearticulate structures of male power and privilege. I have given myself that task, and I am finding my own pace, although it is a constant struggle not only with the patriarchal society we live in but also with the power in our hands as parents. I embrace that honour every day. Such parenting does not consist of an adopted set of norms of conduct but rather consistently asking ethical questions about how to live better in a context where inequality thrives. How do we nurture our son in a way that teaches him to build relationships with others on the firm idea that everyone is equal? Certainly, a child will have a more loving and closer bond and relationship in a family where his or her rights are respected and fulfilled. In such a setting, the wellbeing of the child is being attended to, which enables him or her to form positive, loving, and communal ties.

Mothering from a Distance: Contesting the Notions of Good Mothering

In exploring the process of being a feminist parent, I have found it to be inextricably tied to other aspects of my life. When I reflect on the feminist battles that bubbled up into my life before I even knew how to label it, they were always about claiming my identity and deciding on what kind of person I wanted to be outside of the mother and wife roles. I wanted an identity beyond wife and mother. It followed that I had my undergraduate and master's degree and started my career soon after. Then I got married at twenty-four to my amazing and extremely supportive husband. At twenty-five, I gave birth to my amazing son.

My feminist commitments in raising my son also mean ensuring that I am my full self. As a result, I enrolled into a PhD program in the U.S. and am doing research in Africa. I have thoughts, goals, and ideas unrelated to my role as a mother, such as seeing myself as an individual other than Mahy's mother. These choices are tough ones, but as a family, we continuously find ways to make it work. Realizing that being immigrants living in the diaspora means parenting in isolation from our extended family and without adequate social support, we decided to send our son to his grandparents in the Gambia, which was an opportunity for him to spend time knowing the culture, bonding with relatives, and discovering his roots. Despite the hardships, we all turned out well.

Nonetheless, with this decision, I began to realize what I already knew: that my nontraditional motherhood journey questions the very basic tenets of the ideology of the mother that is embedded in the society I was raised in. Over the years, I have heard countless repetitions and variations of the question "How can you be away from your son?" This is usually followed by judgmental statements: "I cannot imagine myself doing that," "How I wish I have your strength to do what you did," and so on and so forth. Each statement tries to label me as a selfish mother, basically one who is not really a mother at all. They wonder how a loving mother could choose to leave their child behind to pursue an educational opportunity, which is a choice many men make, yet there are no judgments. An absent mother is not socially approved of.

My process of mothering is complicated by cross-cultural constructions of motherhood roles and my own perceptions of being physically away from my son, which leads to feelings of guilt—am I doing what is right? However, I like to believe that I am not doing anything that will be inherently damaging to my son. Although I was already empowered, a doctorate degree means more: it means I may be better able to take care of and protect my son (or other children in the future). I do hope that a well-rounded, fulfilled mother makes for a happy child.

Parenting from a distance is no easy task. It requires focus and additional commitment. We ensure that we remain interested and involved in our child's life. We make it a point to know the names of adults or children that he interacts with—his teachers, classmates, or friends. We FaceTime with him regularly to have real-time conversations. It also helps that at five years old he can pick up his grandparents' phone and give us a call by himself. In doing so, we keep abreast of our child's activities and, at the same time, achieve a certain level of familiarity and intimacy. This is not to downplay the emotional tensions associated with his being far away. In pursuing my dreams, I am missing my son's first swimming lessons as well as story time.

We made the decision to ask a lot of people to help us; our families do help a lot. I hope our son knows that we are decent parents. Despite the pain of separation, I feel like my child will benefit from knowing that his mother lived her best life and pursued her dreams.

Practicing Feminist Parenting

Practicing feminist parenting to me is about teaching my son how to become the kind of person who would be willing to speak up against sexism. Practically, this has meant teaching him to question language, labels, and stereotypes. For example, whilst riding to daycare over the holidays when he visited the U.S., my son made an elephant noise which I tried to make but failed miserably. Then he said, "Only boys can," words that created a straight up feminist nightmare for me. I was in shock, but I was not quick to critique; instead, I listened to him explain why he thought so, since this was an opportunity for retooling the gender stereotype he had picked up from other kids. It was also an opening for a conversation, in which I was able explore and ask him questions to understand his thinking. I was able to explain that it was not about being a girl or a boy. I am certain that this is not a one-off event, as I envisage my son's journey will be as messy as mine still is—or even messier because the times are different and radically becoming more divergent. We are in for a good and long journey, if life permits.

My son is only five years old, but how he is socialized and what behaviours we (my husband and I) exhibit in the house can influence his outlook of what being a man or woman is. Actions speak louder than words. Domestic chores are for both my husband and me to do. We cook and do laundry together, and whoever is free washes the dishes. I make sure my son helps too. "Cooking, washing and doing the domestic chores are not the work of the girl or woman only," I always tell my son. He now attempts to wash the dishes or mop the floor. He is particularly at ease using the traditional wooden mortar and pestle to grind ginger and spices. We also take turns with our son's bedtime routine, although, he usually prefers his dad, since I am the one reminding him about bedtime.

As parents, we are also able to present our son with the opportunity to have a different view about female figures in his TV shows. We encourage him to watch shows that signify strength and adventure regardless of the gender of the characters. His favourite show is *Dora the Explorer*, which features the adventures of a seven-year-old American girl of Indigenous Mexican heritage. My son absolutely adores the quests she undertakes and the places she goes to. His second favourite show is *Go, Diego, Go*, which is about the adventures of Diego, who loves nature and animals and is close kin of Dora. I hope we will get him to be interested in and to watch more gender-balanced content in the future.

Being in the Gambia allows him to enjoy the traditions that we did growing up, including *poti'nyebeh*, a game played outside on the street, singing and dancing, and storytelling by his grandparents and aunties. One of the folktales that he absolutely loves, and is one of the country's most popular, is *Kumba-Am-Ndeye and Kumba-Amul-Ndeye*—a story of two stepsisters who take a magical journey to wash a calabash in a faraway sea. The outcome of each girl's trek depends on her acts of kindness, selfishness, wisdom, and love. Folktales told in the local languages are a huge part of how my son learns more about Gambian history and culture, while imparting him with the moral lessons, which are being handed from one generation to the next. It teaches him that the old should be treated with respect and that strangers should be received hospitably. However, I am also acutely aware that some of these folktales reinforce gender stereotypes, including notions around girls being obedient and polite and boys being brave. By working more actively to share stories about women and girls, both now and as he matures into an adult, we hope that it will help him learn to be respectful and have a worldview centred on equality.

Reflecting on my mothering journey also reminds me of how I make space for solidarity, support, and friendship. For example, the Seattle Feminist Collective's reading group and the Fierce Fabulous Feminist First Fridays have been an amazing space for resisting oppression and reclaiming power. The concept and practice of community is central and germane to the feminist movement and discourse. My life and feminism have been truly affected by my friends all around the world, mostly working professionals doing the work of feminism as well as being mothers and wives. It is truly important to have friends who you can share and connect with because they have been there. My friends, sisters, and mentors are constant reminder for me of our shared day-to-day practice of feminist parenting through our actions and words. We share our joys and challenges of raising boys and how we can continually strive to find fulfillment in our personal and professional lives. It is how we ask more of ourselves.

Conclusion

Through my practice of mothering as an African feminist, I reshape traditional conceptualizations of motherhood through my own journey, which necessitates a more flexible view of what it means to be a good mother. The relationship between being a woman and performing my mothering role from a distance shows that the complexity of motherhood is continually shaped by several factors, including cultural norms, genders roles, as well as social and economic conditions. As a feminist, and more importantly as a feminist parent, I must reaffirm and celebrate the mantra that the personal is truly inviolably political. I hope that my feminist mothering can contribute to social change and to the dismantling of the systems of oppression. Here's to creating feminist opportunities for raising sons who are confident, free to pursue their dreams, and value equality.

Chapter 7

A Muslim Feminist Mother

Astou Ka

Introduction

Having grown up in a patriarchal society, many of my aspirations as a young girl were always centred on getting married, having a family, and catering to my husband and children as dictated by Senegalese culture. I was raised to be ready for marriage and motherhood. I was raised to be a so-called real woman, meaning I had to know how to cook, clean (not only for myself but for my brothers as well), and wash my own clothes. My brothers never had to lift a finger and were free to go play whenever they pleased. I grew up hearing everyone around me say "*Taaru jigen moy sëy*" (i.e., the importance of a woman in society is determined by her marital status). And once marital status is attained, a real woman is expected to not only bear children but always seek to please her man through the art of *jonge* (i.e., always seeking new and improved ways to make her man happy) and be an expert in the art of what we call "*muñ*" (i.e., to bear the burden of whatever ill treatment came her way at the hands of her husband). A woman was to suffer at the hands of her man and never complain because it was her duty to bear the burden. A man was at liberty to do whatever he pleased—no matter whether it was cheating (this had to be expected because after all it is in his nature) or being violent, unaffectionate, or lazy. A woman had to endure it if she ever hoped to have good, successful children in the future. After all, *Ligeey u ndey, añup doom* (i.e. a child will only eat the fruits of his or her mother's labour in the marital home). These constructs were the product of a misogynistic culture and its traditions, which more often than not are falsely attributed to religion (be it Christianity, Islam, or other traditional African religions). From an Islamic standpoint, these misogynistic social constructs were reinforced daily by what I would later come to understand as religiously ignorant, misogynistic, and self-serving imams. As a young Senegalese Muslim (mostly by upbringing at the time and not by choice), these misogynistic views were deeply disturbing to me and led to a long journey into my adulthood of trying to find out and understand on my own the positions of Islam on women's issues. My feminism is deeply influenced by Islam; the two (my Islam and my feminism) have been reconciled, and they have shaped the woman and mother I am today. In this chapter, I take the reader through my journey for the search and discovery of a feminist Islam and how this has influenced my views as a Muslim feminist mother.

Search

I was born and raised in Senegal, a West African nation of about 10 million people, where Muslims, Christians, and other minority religions coexist in peace and brotherhood. It is also a patriarchal and misogynistic society in many aspects by tradition and culture; it is a society where the belief of women's inferiority and second-class citizenship is deeply ingrained in everyone, regardless of religion. Although relative importance is given to women because of their status as child bearers, they are still treated as second-class citizens. In rural Senegal, for example, boys are schooled, whereas girls are expected to help around the home, get married (sometimes very young), and cater to their husbands and bear children. In nonrural Senegal, even if girls are schooled, they are still trained to be home makers as well as husband pleasers. When it comes to women, everything in Senegalese society is centered on pleasing, catering, and obeying men. At a young age, girls are taught the art of submitting to their husband's every single desire. Girls and boys grow up watching their mothers, more often than not, suffer in loveless marriages, devoid of respect and dignity. Those same women will not only accept their dire situations but still strive to fulfill and/or anticipate their husbands' every single wish and whim; these same women will teach their children that such treatment is acceptable. Children grow up being taught and believing that a woman's pride is in achieving her husband's (and his family's) approval and having her praises sung because she suffered through the unthinkable. In this majority Muslim nation, polygamy is allowed, and Muslim girls are taught to expect it, to accept it, and, once in it, to compete for the man's attention at any cost. Boys are taught it is okay to be married and to step out of the marriage as often as they'd like (it is expected in fact). I can remember that even as a child and then teenager, I found this treatment of women around me quite appalling.

I could not comprehend why I, as a girl, had to spend my after-school hours helping around the house while my brothers were allowed to go out and play; I could not comprehend why I had to be quiet and not voice my opinions when my brothers were encouraged to do so; I could not comprehend why my sisters and female cousins on their wedding days were advised to not even think about divorcing and/or coming back to the family home, no matter how bad their marriages were; they had to *muñ*. I was taught that not only did I have to accept this fate but that I also had to act accordingly in order to be seen as a good woman; I was expected to teach this to my children. To make matters worse, Senegalese imams and Muslim scholars cemented this by claiming that Islam taught as much. As a Muslim teenager, this was disturbing to say the least. As such, when I came to the United States, after high school, in the early 2000s, I made it a point to learn about Islam and understand this religion I was born into. One thing you will discover in many majority Muslim countries is that more often than not people who are born into religion perform the prescribed rituals without really understanding the religion they claim as theirs; they blindly follow what others interpret for them to be Islam. Senegal is no exception. I was taught how to pray, fast, and do other rituals. I was taught to recite the Qur'an in Arabic without understanding a single word that was being uttered. As a result, during my college days in a Catholic Jesuit school, although I majored in finance, many of my elective classes were about understanding Islam (yes, at a Catholic Jesuit University!); this was in addition to classes I took at my local mosque, the Internet searches I personally conducted, as well as the many debates I had with other Muslim friends and classmates. I learned a lot during this investigative period. But my enlightenment, if you will, occurred while taking a women in Islam class at Santa Clara University, taught by a Sudanese-American woman, whose name I cannot presently recall. One of the accompanying books of that class was "*Believing Women*" *in Islam: Unreading Patriarchal Interpretations of the Qur'an* by Asma Barlas, a professor of politics at Ithaca College. Barlas says that "Non-Muslims point to the subjugation of women that occurs in many Muslim countries, especially those that claim to be 'Islamic,' while Muslims read the Qur'an in ways that seem to justify sexual oppression, inequality, and patriarchy" (Barlas, back cover). What Professor Barlas did for me was to "develop a believer's reading of the Qur'an that demonstrates the radically egalitarian and antipatriarchal nature of its teachings" (Barlas, back cover).

Discovery

I have discovered and learned that what Islam preaches is not inequality or the subjugation of women; rather, it preaches for equity between the two sexes—equity in that there are notable differences between men and women in various aspects. For example, men and women are made differently physically, physiologically, and emotionally, and, as such, they play different roles in society to mutually complement one another. For example, women menstruate, and men don't; that's a fact. Women can carry and bear children, men don't; that's a fact. More often than not, women are more nurturing, caring, and compassionate than men; that's a fact. Men are generally physically stronger than women because of hormones; that's a fact. Now, does this mean that one is superior to the other? No! Just that they are made differently; that's it. The fact that men deserve respect, worship, and catering because of their perceived physical and emotional strength is not an Islamic construct; rather, it is a sociocultural construct strengthened by "misogynistic readings/interpretations of the Qur'an derived not from the Qur'an, but from attempts by Muslim exegetes and Qur'an commentators to legitimize actual usage of their own day by interpreting it in great detail into the Holy Book" (Barlas 8). As Professor Barlas points out, the "Qur'an appoints men and women as each other's *Awliya*, or mutual protectors (Qur'an 9:71), which it could not do if men were in fact superior to women and their 'managers'" (Barlas 186). Although this chapter does not have the space to deeply dive into misogynistic interpretations of the Qur'an, I will just provide one example. In Islam, God is genderless, yet in all interpretations of the Qur'an, God, or Allah, is referred to as a "He." In fact, the word

"Allah," which God has asked Muslims to refer to as "Him," is neither feminine nor masculine, yet all Muslims refer to *Allah* as "He."

The status of women, especially mothers, is high in Islam. This narration of the Prophet Muhammad (peace and blessings be upon him) is an illustration:

> A man came to the Prophet and said, "O Messenger of God! Who among the people is the worthiest of my good companionship?" The Prophet (PBUH) said: Your mother. The man said, "Then who?" The Prophet said: Then your mother. The man further asked, "Then who?" The Prophet said: Then your mother. The man asked again, "Then who?" The Prophet said: Then your father." (Islam Celebrates Women)

The Prophet (peace and blessings be upon him), here, highlights the importance of the mother over the father by repeating "your mother" three times and then saying "your father" once in response to the man's question. Additionally, per the Prophet (peace and blessings be upon him): "Paradise is at the feet of the mother."

A Muslim Feminist Mother

What kind of a feminist am I? I am a feminist whose views are deeply influenced by Islam in that I believe in equity. I don't believe in the superiority of one sex over another; however; in Islam, the "rights and responsibilities of a woman are equal to those of a man, but they are not necessarily identical with them. Equality and sameness are two quite different things. This difference is understandable because man and woman are not identical, but they are created equals" (Abdul-Ati). As such, I am not the feminist who will take off her bra in protest against a symbol of oppression or show my equality to men; I recognize I was made as a woman, with breasts, and I will do anything I can to slow down gravity from pulling them down to my knees. The distinction between equality and sameness is important. Equality is desirable, just, and fair, but sameness is not. People are not created identical, but they are created as equals. What I try to teach to my boys is that there is no ground to assume that a woman is less important than a man just because her rights are not identically the same as his. The fact that Islam gives her equal rights—but not identical—shows that it takes married in 1990 in Lawrence, Kansas—where I had gone to university.

My husband is named Penangnini, which means, "What does it take to live together in peace?" What a big question for him to carry throughout life! Tagbana by ethnicity, he grew up in Katiola, a little north of Cote d'Ivoire's second largest city of Bouake. He grew up among the Baoulé people—who migrated to the area from present-day Ghana—and the Dioula, who migrated from the north and spread Dioula as a trading language. People mixed and spoke one another's languages. Being multicultural and multilingual was and still is a way of life.

I wonder if my husband's question about more natural birth control methods came from his proximity to his grandmother, Aya, a midwife and herbalist. Growing up, he followed her to people's homes where she "caught babies"; he saw how she massaged newborns and shared her energy with them. He saw people from near and far stopping by the compound to consult his grandmother who proposed appropriate remedies for their ailments. Was Grandma Aya somehow present as we gave birth to two of her descendants?

Our first child came into the world in a one-bedroom student-housing apartment in Iowa City. We had moved there for my husband to pursue a master's degree in communications. I worked at the Center for International and Comparative Studies. My husband made dinner one evening, and we ate after I returned from the office. The contractions began shortly thereafter.

The midwife asked on the phone if she had time to renew her driver's license and then head to our place. I responded that, as a still inexperienced birther and a mother-to-be, I was not well qualified to assess and advise in that regard. She sent the assistant midwife, who during the birthing process coached my husband to be useful by keeping a warm washcloth on my lower back. Each time he left to warm the cloth, I cried out that my back hurt. My husband and I demonstrated how birth control, birth itself, and the later raising of children are all shared responsibilities.

When the assistant midwife (because the midwife had still not arrived) put our child face down on my chest, with the umbilical cord still attached, none of us thought about whether this beautiful being with pink skin and tufts of black hair was a boy or a girl. We were just relieved, filled with joy, grateful, and in admiration.

Secretly, I desired a daughter, as I thought I knew more about girls and would know how to raise one. "What would I do with a boy? How would I relate?" I often asked myself. Eventually, the assistant midwife investigated and mentioned that our baby was a girl. That is when we knew she would be called Aya Sophia, the names of her parents' paternal grandmothers.

My husband wanted to honour his grandmother, Missa Aya, who had seen him grow up in Katiola, by naming our daughter after her. My mother-in-law thought we were not going back far enough, generationally, with "Aya," but she acquiesced. Aya, in Baoulé, means "girl born on Friday." Although our Aya was born on a Saturday, she started making her way into the world on a Friday. Sophia was the name of my grandmother who, with her husband, raised my father and his two older brothers and three older sisters on a farm in eastern Kansas.

At about 5:00 p.m. on the day of Aya's birth, we heard a knock on the door. The midwife, who had arrived a few minutes earlier, answered the door, and we heard, "Trick or Treat." Yes, it was October 31—the day Halloween is celebrated in the United States. We felt that our newborn daughter had been well greeted by youngsters from the neighbourhood. The midwife proceeded to put a sign on the door: Just Had a Baby, Please Come Back Next Year.

I did not know, or had forgotten, about afterbirth. My husband cut the umbilical cord and held Aya while the midwife and her assistant got me up and instructed me to squat. Later that evening or the next day, my husband took a spade and the bin with the placenta and walked to the nearby park filled with walking trails and trees. When he came back, he explained that it was not easy at all to dig into the cold earth. I got the impression he might not be in a hurry to bury another placenta. I am sure that the tree he dug beneath is growing well.

Girlfriends of mine had organized a shower for me about a month before Aya was born. We had requested that guests bring books for the baby. I was appreciative. However, in reviewing the books, my husband and I noted how they predominantly featured white characters. We felt this would be problematic and made a point to diversify our library going forwards.

About twenty months after the birth of Aya, my husband and I were ready to give birth to our second child. We headed to the hospital—because a homebirth was not covered by insurance. We felt we had knowledge and experience this time around and could manage a natural birth, even at the hospital. Staff at the birthing ward assigned us a nurse who had accompanied many homebirths. I render homage to her. Because we declined the use of a sonogram, while I stood, she got down on her knees to check the heartbeat of the baby with a stethoscope and charted it out on paper by hand.

As soon as our baby cleared the birth canal, the midwife-nurse declared, in the rather classic fashion, "It's a boy!" I understood how thrilled my husband was when I saw him spontaneously hug the messenger while our son suckled without restraint at my breast. I too was happy.

Later, a hospital staff member declared, "Mrs. Toure, you are the only woman we have ever seen at University Hospitals and Clinics not belted down to the bed to be monitored via screens at the reception." I was distressed to learn in the medical world what is often visited unquestionably upon people.

Our son was named Gninnanhoyan by my mother-in-law, which means, "God sees us" or "God sees everything." Later in life, he gained the middle name of Patrick, which we added to his birth certificate. After observing with him a Taekwondo class while he was in primary school, we asked, "Do you want to join the class?" He responded emphatically, "No. The maître calls the name of each student at the beginning of class. He would never be able to pronounce my name." Tagbana names are indeed not that easy, even for Ivorians. They are the beginning of a thought, of a sentence. People sometimes have the nerve to ask for nicknames in their place. Today, however, Patrick bears his first name of Gninnanhoyan with pride.

We moved to Cote d'Ivoire when Aya was two-and-a-half years old, and Gninnanhoyan was still nursing. After a month, I returned to the United States to continue my work at the University of Iowa, while my husband stayed with the children and looked for work. Our son was suddenly severed from the breast one day at the airport. My husband has not forgotten those days and nights of trying to comfort him, and I have not forgotten how I finally learned to stop the flow of milk with the application of ice.

In the beginning, my husband stayed with the children at his mother's place in Bouake in the middle of the country. My mother-in-law looked after the children during the day. Unlike their cousins born in the capital city of Abidjan, our children spoke Tagbana fluently with their grandmother. My husband had spoken only in his mother tongue with them since the day they were born. He would say: "*Manan nan glan*" ("I love you, one person"); "*Ye nan glan*" ("I love you, several people"); and "*Nan pili ye nan nan glan*" ("I love you, my children"). Aya and Gninnanhoyan went in a reddish Renault 4 taxi to school at the *Grande Cathédrale* in Bouake, with their elder cousin Soutcho Lydie. Soutcho means "girl born on Saturday" in Tagbana.

After about six months, my husband had already found a job, and I moved to Cote d'Ivoire and found a job in the capital city of Abidjan. I traveled by bus every two weeks to Bouake to see the family. One Sunday when I was ready to return to Abidjan, Aya said, "Goodbye, Auntie." That is when I discussed things with my husband, and we decided we would all live together in Abidjan.

By the time Aya was five and starting kindergarten (*grande section*) in Abidjan, she and Gninnanhoyan attended *Groupe Scolaire Jacques Prévert*. One Saturday after school, we ate lunch and began reviewing vocabulary in French. Aya's class was studying the names of the parts of the body. We made flash cards together, and I lay on the tiled living room floor in our neighbourhood of Attoban. Gninnanhoyan gave the flashcards one by one to Aya, and I coached her when she was not quite sure whether to place one on my heart, hand, or forehead.

My husband came home and asked what we were doing and said we should take studying seriously. We gathered up the cards, and he sat with Aya, Gninnanhoyan, and their schoolbooks at the low round wooden children's table with six chairs, each painted a different colour. I knew the children would learn that there is no one way to do something.

One Christmas, Aya, now about eight years old, put a note under the tree: "Dear Santa, I am asking for anything but a book." We didn't really do gifts much, and Aya knew what they were if we did, but I surprised her, and myself, on about her ninth birthday. We had just moved to Bamako, in Mali, for the new school year, and she invited girls and boys from her class over to our rented house in the ACI2000 neighbourhood. In honour of her Halloween birthday, we carved with her guests jack-o-lanterns from watermelons, which were in season. We took them up to the flat roof of the house before sunset, with one candle in each.

While waiting for nightfall, Aya unwrapped a present I had bought her. She was astounded to see the picture of a baby stroller for a doll on the box. She couldn't believe her eyes and thought for sure there was something else inside. "Mom, you would never get me a stroller," she insisted, looking up at me with big questioning eyes. I had not been drawn to dolls as a child and could not fathom that my daughter could be. She enjoyed playing with that stroller. When we still lived in Iowa City, she would tie a doll to her back and follow me out the apartment door and down the stairs to the clothesline to hang the laundry out to dry. I often attached her brother to my back with a *pagne* (a wrapper made from a two-metre piece of African-print fabric) because it freed up my hands and comforted him, and I realized she was imitating me.

My husband took the children to the doctor at times if they were ailing. When he came home, I asked all the details about the prescription and the medicines. He replied, "If you want to give the children their medicine as prescribed by the doctor, then let me know. I will let you do it." I realized I should not interfere but simply trust him. He also helped the children with their baths. He was the one who gently nursed them if they scraped a knee and needed tender loving care and a Band-Aid. I think that if all men had the opportunity to demonstrate their tenderness, we would have more peace in the world. Sometimes my husband expressed his impatience with me about reading to the children before bed: "I am the one who has to get them to bed. And then you cuddle up with them to read and make me look like the disciplinarian." We constantly negotiated how to parent.

We did not parent on our own or on one continent. During school vacations, Aya and Gninnanhoyan and sometimes Soutcho flew as "unaccompanied minors" to Kanas City to be with their grandparents. They also spent time on the coast in southern New Jersey with my sister and brother-in-law, who still take pride in parenting them: "They are at home with us. We so enjoy biking and kayaking with them. We taught them how to drive a stick shift!"

In preparing to write this essay from Nairobi, Kenya, where my husband and I now live, I wrote on WhatsApp to ask Aya, Gninnanhoyan, and Soutcho, who are all in their twenties and living in Washington DC, if I am indeed a feminist parent.

Aya Sophia responded:

This depends on how one defines feminism, but here are a few examples. I think you've taught us to respect ourselves and others. This is important especially in this day and age where respect does not seem to be taught equally. Part of respecting oneself and others is also standing up for yourself (and others). Chores were distributed equally, not based on sex. Freedom and encouragement to think critically and make decisions for oneself were encouraged. Let me know if you want more (specific examples). I'll keep thinking about it :).

Gninnanhoyan Patrick responded:

If we watched TV, you asked questions about why no women were included in certain discussions or why women were portrayed in certain ways. When I played video games with my friends, you sat beside us and asked questions about what was going on—questions that made us stop and think. You explained things from a woman's perspective. You talked with us about sex and stressed respect and safety.

Soutcho Lydie responded:

Based on my definition of feminism, I think you are a feminist parent. In addition to what Aya and Patrick said, I will say that you encourage us to speak up, to affirm ourselves. For example, you often ask us to share about our day, what we learned, what we did for ourselves, and what we did for others. Also, you taught us how to take care of and protect ourselves to avoid harassment. We shouldn't think that we are inferior to others. If something is not right, we should speak our minds. I think you are more than a feminist. You are a powerful woman who is always positive no matter what. You are full of and spread joy all around you. I really admire that in you! Hope this explains a bit why you are a feminist parent. I hope I have a good understanding of the topic.

When my nieces and nephews in Cote d'Ivoire, including Soutcho, started calling me Mamma, it bothered me quite a bit. I thought, "I have enough children to worry about and do not need more worries." However, living in West Africa, I became accustomed to being Mamma for more than my birth children, and our children have been parented by more than their birth parents because there is a sense of responsibility in the community at large for raising children.

When Soutcho lived with us for a few years in Abidjan, Aya and Patrick's solidarity with her was impressive. When we went to get bikes, they insisted, "Don't forget Soutcho." Only once did I see some jealousy.

mine in what ways the strength of sociocultural norms shaped our struggles to show our children that they can and should question existing hierarchies of power. We count on them to do their part to reshape habits, relationships and societal institutions.

Chapter 9

"A Young Woman's Voice Does Not Break, It Grows firmer"[1]

Rama Salla Dieng

I will tell you, my daughter
of your worth
not your beauty
every day. (your beauty is a given. every being is born beautiful)
knowing your worth
can save your life.
raising you on beauty alone
you will be starved.
you will be raw.
you will be weak.
easy clay.
always in need of someone telling you how beautiful you are.

—emotional nutrition

nayyirah waheed—salt.

In this chapter, I first discuss what being a feminist means to me and the dreams and visions I had prior to becoming a parent as a young woman who wanted to have it all. I will then focus on what my daughter's arrival has meant and what has changed or been challenged. Finally, I share my experience about the dilemmas and compromises of (r)evolutionary love, dealing with grief and the healing and life-transforming potential of telling and sharing our diverse narratives of feminist parenting and re-creating solidarities that were eroded by conjugated patriarchies. I use an intersectional approach as per Crenshaw's use of the term: "Because the intersectional experience is greater than the sum of racism and sexism, any analysis that does not take intersectionality into account cannot sufficiently address the particular manner in which Black women are subordinated" (40). This allows me to focus both on my intersecting vulnerabilities and my intersectional privilege (Cho et al).

I Did Not Have to Decide to Become a Feminist: Life Happened

I have not always wanted to be somebody's wife or life partner. Or a mother. I was born and raised in Senegal in a family of five girls, and one boy, who was also the last child. My parents kept trying for a boy until he was born. In a society valuing boys over girls, no wonder my parents chose the name "*Amine*" for him: a prayer answered in Arabic. My sisters and I were very close friends. This is where my first ideas of sorority and solidarity were forged as well as the belief that we shared a common life experience.

In addition, all my education—primary and secondary—was spent in all-girls schools. My family is not rich, but we have never lacked anything. I was quite a tomboy; I practiced karate, football, and other physical sports, such as "*au-drapeau*" in the streets with my friends (like in the picture below—you do not need to know where I am: I am all of them).

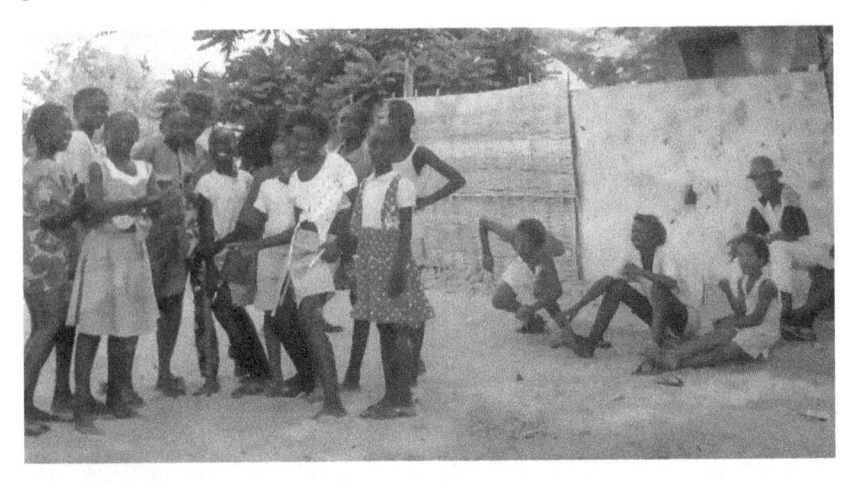

I played sports until my mother decided it was time for my older sister and me to start learning how to cook and take care of a house—to learn to be wife material. We were in secondary school then. Fortunately, my little sister was allowed to pursue karate classes, and she even ended up with a black belt. As for my brother, he never experienced any such restrictions or preoccupations; he did not experience curfew as we did, his male privilege protected him from that.

As for me, though very calm and reserved, I remember at around ten years old having a tough fight with an older male childhood friend because he had said "girls are stupid." I calmly waited until we arrived in a quiet street under construction and full of tar, and then politely asked him, "Can you please repeat what you said earlier." He did. I fought him and sat on him telling him, "Next time, think twice before saying stupid things," and I covered his face with tar. Other than my early feminism and quarrelsome nature, I was a shy bookworm who loved writing short stories and poems in her mathematics book for the entire class to read. I also wore a veil for three years, not only for religious reasons but also as a way of protecting my new femininity and learning to deal with it, after past experiences of abuse.

I left Senegal at the age of eighteen to pursue higher education in France. Being far away from my sisters, as well as being the only member of my family to be abroad, came with a dose of responsibilities and duties; my parents did not spare any occasion to remind me that I am from a "very honourable" family and that I should keep behaving in a way that would not bring shame to them. During my third year of study, I learned that my father had married a second wife. For him, Islam allowed him to marry up to four wives. My mother accepted this because of i) religion, ii) love, and iii) culture. I did not take it well, hence family 'mediation'. After all, the self-nominated mediators asked, who was I to want to be consulted on an issue that was only the business of my two parents? Faced with so many mixed feelings and above all rage, uncontrollable rage, I would write long letters to my mother and other long letters expressing my hate of the double standards of the hypocritical society in which we were raised—one that only knew how to make women seem small. I decided to contribute in an anthology on polygamy, which gave voice to people living in a polygamist household and who most of the time did not make the decision to live that life. I convinced my mother to write a piece, too. I think it helped us both to move ahead, with our scars. Writing became a way for me to take care of myself and of my feelings. To talk back. I did not know Audre Lorde then. But I was echoing what she once said: "what is most important to me must be spoken, made verbal, and shared, even at the risk of having it bruised or misunderstood" (Lorde).

Up to that moment, I viewed my father as a feminist. He empowered us, his daughters and his boy, constantly. He invested in our education and encouraged all our creative passions. I have now made peace with the fact that his polygamy was his choice of life and have learned not to throw the baby out with the bathwater. My father was still loving and caring; he still inspires me on many other levels. But these family experiences created a deeper consciousness of my gender and influenced the choices I would make immediately after. Change city. Change university. Find a job. Be financially autonomous. Write a novel. Have it published. Change my course of studies. Focus on my studies. Make my own decisions. Own them. I started reading the works of African feminists and the work of other African women writers. I also started writing more and more and was glad to find out I was standing on the shoulders of giants.

(Not) Teaching My Mother How to Give Birth[2]

After finishing my studies, I returned to Senegal to work there despite starting a relationship with my now husband. It mattered to me that I work in my own area of specialization after so many years of studies, and it mattered to him to resume his studies. Then my older sister got married, followed by my younger sister. My now husband and I were still dating. I became the focus of my entourage and especially that of my mother. I was still living at home at that age, not only because most unmarried women did but because I wanted to spend time with my family after so many years abroad. For many years, I kept teasing my mother: "you and I will stay in the house after you marry everyone else away." Every day was about resisting her sarcastic comments: "menopause is not far away you know" or "a job is not a husband."

My mother's comments were based on a culture according to which "*taaru jigeen sëy la*," or "the beauty of a woman lies in marriage." This widespread belief makes it so difficult for single women, whereas single men are not subjugated to any form of pressure or social surveillance.

No matter what her professional achievements are, or whether she wished at all to be married, a woman's respectability and her social status depend on her getting married and showing she is able to produce children, preferably males ones, for society.

With my return after my studies, I got involved with an organization focusing on young women's rights. In fact, the year of my return to Senegal coincided with the adoption of the gender parity law, which required political parties to ensure that at least half their candidates in local and national elections are women. This allowed Senegal to rank at seventh place worldwide in 2017 and second in Africa after Rwanda. The country is predominantly Muslim but is renowned for its secularism and prides itself on its decades of peace and security. I, for instance, grew up as a Muslim but went to a Catholic school. Yet my country is also one whose criminal code prohibits abortion except when undertaken to save the pregnant woman's life; moreover, LGBT rights are not protected. Homosexual acts are defined as "acts against nature" and are punishable by up to five years imprisonment. All of this makes Senegal a country of contradictions, where patriarchy today is the legacy not only of French colonization, but also of Islam and its strictures, which were also imported to West Africa. All of these kinds of patriarchy collude with culture to subjugate women and younger men. Yet these versions of culture (and religion) are mostly a legacy of colonialism, which used religion and different tools, such as taxation, to divide and rule (some call it "govern") while reengineering gender identities, family roles, and, hence, domestic power dynamics.

Although this chapter is not primarily about how coloniality has survived colonialism, I think it is worth giving an example. Even though matrilineal societies are often patriarchal in specific ways, they also contain empowering dimensions: in matriarchal groups, such as the Sereer, the links between one's mother's brother and sister and their child are close, and they can inherit from the maternal uncle. However, matrilineal groups (descent through the mother's line, such as in the Sereer ethnic group) or bilineal groups (descent through both the mother's and father's line, such as in the Wolof ethnic group) are becoming more and more patrilineal (descent through the father's line, such as in the Pulaar-Fulani ethnic group) (Diop). This is important because whereas patrilineal groups are almost always patriarchal—power and descent converge—the same cannot be said for matrilineal

Becoming a Mother

Just after our marriage, we moved to London, I from Senegal and he from France, after leaving his job. Soon after, our families started pressuring us again, this time, to have a child. We resisted. I was studying, and he was just starting his career after finishing his studies. We decided that we clearly were not ready. A few years after the wedding, the situation became worse with people within our entourage even insinuating that I (not him) had health or fertility issues and that we should consult a doctor. We decided not to pay any attention. He was even the first to cut short such conversations and questioning, as it was no one else's business.

Many months after, we decided we were ready to have a child. This was in the first year of my PhD. I remember wanting to have it all in my early twenties: pursuing my writing, starting my doctoral studies, being more financially autonomous, and then, maybe, having a child. I did not publish a second novel, although I was still writing, but all the rest happened in that exact order. We thought then that it was the best time, as I could do my fieldwork while benefiting from the support of my family in Senegal and I could write from anywhere, as my type of studies was part time.

I became pregnant immediately after we started trying, and I can remember knowing so intimately the exact moment I felt pregnant, despite the five or six pregnancy tests telling me otherwise. I kept buying them until one test indicated that I was one to two weeks pregnant a few days later.

Three months into the pregnancy, after knowing the sex of our baby, I wrote a letter to her promising to guide her into this world while remaining true to ourselves. Our families, though in Senegal, started making a lot of recommendations: I should cover my body and my head, avoid working at certain times (before 7:00 a.m., between 1:00 pm and 2:00 p.m. and after 7:00 p.m.) to avoid the "evil eye," and be more obedient to my husband because the character of my future child and her destiny depended on my being a good wife. This reminded me of my many readings about how in my culture, the uterine descent or mother's line is said to transmit blood (*dereet*), character (*jikko*), and flesh (*suux*) to the progeny, while the patrilineal descent determines the nerves (*siditt*), the bones (*yax*), and courage (*fit*) (Diagne; Diop). If both descents are important, the matriline is, in reality, given more significance because it is supposed to determine the qualities of the children through the mother's milk (*meen*). To illustrate this, only the matrikin is said to permit the transmission of witchcraft (*ndëmm*) to the offspring; also, the success of the children is said to depend on the mother's behaviour as illustrated by many Wolof proverbs, such as "*ligeeyu ndey, añup doom*" ("a mother's work is lunch for her children"). This saying means that women who endure their marriage will have successful children. As for the father's line, it transmits the surname to the child who belongs to the father's family, who is supposed to be responsible for the women and children.

Despite being broke at the time, we wanted a proper naming ceremony for our daughter with a couple of friends. We, however, decided not to follow some of the prescriptions of our ethnic group to name a daughter after her grandfather's sisters. We decided to give her the two first names of our mothers, my middle name (which all our children will bear, if there are others), and her father's surname. This was because I was more attached to my middle name, Rama, than to my father's surname, which I had, nonetheless, kept after our marriage because my religion, Islam, advises that a woman doesn't change her name after marriage.

Throughout my pregnancy, I continued being a whole woman; I explored any facet of life I had interest in and kept my options open. I worked on my PhD project while travelling and working and exercising until my eighth month of pregnancy.

Becoming a Feminist Activist-Scholar Mother: A Young Woman's Voice Does Not Break

Before the pregnancy, we had discussed several times our ideal future. Of course, I wanted to resume my professional life after my doctoral studies, but I had never been very at ease a with fixed nine-to-five job. I enjoyed being a scholar-activist at the same time. However, I did not understand that being a new mother would, in fact, lead to reorganizing all of my other activities around it. Just when I found out I was pregnant, I had launched a series of interviews with scholars, activists, artists, and policymakers on issues of interest to the continent. As an early African researcher geographically based in the United Kingdom, I wanted to initiate a dialogue with other young Africans in the diaspora and on the continent on issues of mutual interest. Did my pregnancy trigger my wish to be more of an activist trying to decolonise and democratise knowledge while abolishing boundaries between policy research and action, and contributing to the legacy we would transmit to the ones yet to come? I don't know. I am still thinking about the role of the intellectual, but it is certainly not a role that only requires thinking without transforming the world(s) we have in common. In my dream feminist future, I would work just a few hours per day to earn a living—the necessary amount to be comfortable. Becoming rich has never been a life objective for me. I was, therefore, also thinking about financial sustainability.

The final week of the pregnancy was fast approaching. After four days of going to the hospital and being returned home, labour finally started on a Tuesday night. After several hours of gas and air, screaming, laughing, and crying, our daughter finally arrived the following day by water birth. This allowed us both to play an active role during the delivery. My husband in particular was the one doing extensive skin-to-skin contact with her while I was sleeping. I was grateful I did not have any stitches; I just felt sleepy and hungry afterwards. The first few days of us returning home were sleepless as well as emotionally and physically exhausting, but we were amazed by her.

After her arrival, life as we knew it was over, as were the certainties and the values my mother inculcated in me. We decided we would invent a new path for our family. And for the two parents we were, our naivety to believe we could be a nice feminist family was a blessing in disguise. The likely scenario for our team was that I would be the main caring parent (I thought I could work on my PhD from home) and he would be the second parent. But then, I realized that was not what I wanted. I did not work hard to start a PhD only to suddenly renounce to everything because of motherhood. We decided to have a child together; we would share the tasks equally. We had several conversations, often stormy, and we finally came to the agreement to share the tasks equally accordingly to financial contribution. I had four days and he one initially because I had a student budget. But I decided it was unfair because of all the emotional and unpaid care work I was also doing when I was at home with her. I started working part time from home when my daughter was sleeping and when I was not working on my research project. As for my husband, he started developing his own projects before we decided to have a child. But with pregnancy, his wish to work for himself and be able to design his own business model and have more flexible working hours became stronger. Therefore, he started to work part time for another company while working on his project the rest of the time. And just after the birth of our daughter, he resigned from his job and started working fulltime on his project with his business partner. He initially started working four days a week and worked from home the rest of the week, when he would be the main carer. Eventually, he started working three days a week away from home and two from home to take care of our daughter while I was at the university library. I reckon we were able to reorganize ourselves and reach our dream parenting balance because of his intersecting privileges (Cho et al): the flexibility of his job came from a firm and carefully designed agreement on what we wanted our parenting our child to resemble.

After welcoming our daughter into this world, we were tired, but little did we know that what we were experiencing at the time was the mildest level of tiredness. Fortunately, a few weeks after our daughter was born, my mother came to London from Senegal to spend a month with us. And with her visit, I rediscovered how being a mother is valued in my society: the massages that are provided to both mother and baby, and the special preparation of the mother's food for her to have the nutrients she and the baby need, and the long hours to rest. Some women even leave the marital house to return to their parents' house to rest and be taken care of. All of which I did not have in London, and even breastfeeding in public is still an issue.

Soon after, with the prospect of resuming my studies after a six-month maternity break, I realized my biggest challenge would be to reconcile my new role of mother with those of expatriate, feminist, passionate wife and lover, resourceful student-researcher, reader, and tireless traveller. I was torn between the refuge-cocoon that I had built since I became a mother and the prospect of returning to a busy life. Also, at the beginning of the adventure of mothering, I was not able to find the precious time I used to have to spend with myself; the sweet solitude that I loved to slip into in order to read, write, feel, meditate, and reflect was only but a memory. When my daughter was sixteen months old, I decided to stop the breastfeeding, and then a few weeks after, we found a nursery place for her. She went three days a week, and each of us had her for one day a week. Since we had found an emotional, social, financial, and love balance after the initial earthquake of parenting, I decided to resume participating in academic conferences, which is an important facet for any researcher (or researcher-to-be). This forced me to familiarize myself with all the logistics behind #PhDoingWhileParenting, and I was struck by a harsh reality: 95 per cent of conference organizers refuse to take care of the additional cost of travelling with a baby, even if she is breastfeeding. Several times, I had to buy her ticket (thankfully only 10 per cent of the price of my ticket), find a babysitter while in London, and arrive a little earlier so that the nanny got to spend time with my little one in my presence for her to get used to being without me (the settling period). During the conferences, I had to escape during lunch and coffee breaks to breastfeed and spend time with my little one.

We decided to resume our respective activities. In March that year, I had to go to Cape Town, South Africa, for a program on leading in public life. From our first interactions, the organizers made it clear that they would not take care of my daughter's ticket but encouraged me to wait until the following year. I refused because I believed mothers are the first leaders in public life, and it was out of the question for me to exclude myself. My husband was able to find a babysitter, thanks to his circle of friends in the Cape area, where he had worked for a while. Imagine the cost of a baby ticket and two weeks of babysitting on a student budget. But I took part anyway, and this program transformed me. But this intensive program was also a marathon. While my daughter was resting well in our hotel room, I went on all-day rounds to breastfeed and spend time with her. I'm proud to have also had an impact on the organizers, as they have decided from now on to take care of the costs for babies (less than one year) of parents who take part in the program—it was not retroactive, though.

After this conference, I went to another trip in Southern Africa. This conference went well, but the return flight was catastrophic, as we were taken off the plane in Lusaka on suspicion of a contagious disease. I was in an unknown country and was forcefully removed from the plane with my baby because I expressed the fear that I might have an allergy after I started itching. Despite finding a bed bug in my clothing, which I showed to the flight attendant, I was taken out of the plane and left with the promise I would be booked another flight if I brought the proof of my fitness to travel. When my colleagues and passengers dared to interrogate why I was taken out for examination, since I had nothing—even a doctor proposed to consult me on board—they were all made to sit down and mind their own business. Then I let my anger explode, which led to the police and security being called, who threatened me to stop filming the scene with my camera and then threatened to separate me from my daughter if I did not leave the Emirates plane. Yes, there it was: Misogynoir! The intersection between racism and sexism to make me—yet another angry black woman who dared to resist and speak up—shut the fuck up!

When I returned to London, I was traumatized. Even the messages of support, sympathy, and encouragement from friends left me with this bitter taste of doubt. Then I resolved: if I let this experience traumatize me, my relationship to parenting, to mothering, and to my social relationships would be transformed forever. I started to firmly agree with Ama Ata Aidoo that "a girl's voice does not break, it grows firmer." Having an academic and a professional life for a Senegalese woman living in Europe, especially in England, has emotional, social, and financial costs, but this is not a reason to systematically refuse invitations or to not ask that the cost of travelling with your little one be covered if you travel with her, as I do. Even if the response is a no, I go anyway because it is important to continue to occupy these spaces and not to exclude myself. And when I do go, I undertake another type of advocacy around why we need to occupy these spaces with our children.

At home, I started talking more to my child about feelings and how to express them and manage them, and to my husband; I voiced my anger whenever I felt it and encouraged them to do the same. I started listening more to his laments and his intersecting vulnerabilities, especially around toxic masculinity, which would constantly judge him because he wanted to be another type of father for his daughter—one that would be more present, express his feelings, and encourage her to respect her opinions and her body and to know that she was enough. This reminded me of an anthology exploring *Fathers and Daughters* relations edited by Ato Quayson. In his chapter *Voyage Round my Daughter* in Quayson's anthology, Simon Gikandi shares the following:

> Stories of fathers and daughters ... are weapons against the stigma that we African men are condemned to bear in our sojourns in the world of the other. We know what this stigma is because we live with it—the unquestioned assumption, irrespective of our

from generation to generation. For instance, I have always admired how in Senegal, women who have just given birth are taken care of. I also from time to time have loved to challenge those who follow any cultural practice simply because that is the way things should be. Therefore, having my mother keep asking me questions about her grandchild getting her ears pierced even after she left must have reawakened my mischievous side. And frankly I had not particularly reflected on those questions and just thought it wasn't a priority, since my schedule on those first months was quite hectic. I must have asked once at the medical centre whether they pierced babies' ears and they answered they did not. Then I might have decided it was not that important. But witnessing the cries of my daughter because I was too much of a coward to say, "No, she will decide when she grows up," left me with the firm decision I would not let such a thing happen again.

Reflecting on how to articulate my resistance, I decided that writing and organizing collectively to amplify parents' voices on feminist parenting was crucial, especially by mobilizing such experiences in the non-Western world. How was it that I saw rarely African and Global South feminists publicly discuss the issue of feminist parenting? Was it because after long, secular struggles to prove they could work outside the house, some of them did not want to return in the private sphere and decided not to reclaim parenting as a prime and fertile political site? Or was it still the old debate between womanism[3] and African and Black feminism(s)? Wasn't there any value of reclaiming anything domestic, since many feminists saw motherhood as one of the principal reasons for women's subjugation to patriarchy: the vile production and reproduction to sustain capitalism(s) and patriarchies? Or was the erasure of African and Global South feminist parents' (and children)'s agency because they needed to be (re)presented as only poor women and girls without any agency—an image dear to the mainstream aid and development industry? All these reflections led me to return to the writings from the non-Western world. From familiarizing myself with the writings of Western feminists such as Adrienne Rich's *Of Women Born,* I then migrated all the way to Chimamanda Ndozi Adichie's *Dear Ijeawele* and Oyèrónké Oyèwùmí's *What Gender Is Motherhood?*. My child was then eight months old. The Feminist Parenting book project has been an adventure for me, and I believe for the other parents involved as well, because the idea came from personal reflections about the way

I wanted to relate to my child—the way I found myself doing it because I am in a heterosexual couple, and the way the outside world is also intervening and sometimes mediating, facilitating, and disrupting my parenting practice. I wanted to know the personal history of every contributing parent and how each understood their story of feminist parenting, including the why and the why not as well as the how and under which circumstances. It was a collective learning process for all of us through the owning, telling, and sharing of our experiences. It has been an adventure.

Passing on Life and Love, Dealing with Grief and Bringing the Village Back In

My older sister, Anta, recently passed away, a few hours after giving birth to her third healthy child. It was not a natural death. It was not an accident. It was medical error. This awakens so many questions for me: how feasible and realistic is conceptualizing feminist futures when women are still dying from giving birth in 2019? This shows how the personal remains political and how the economic is also political. The lack of adequate health infrastructure, as well as the lack of qualified provision of health services, kills. The lack of basic social services kills. Corruption kills. The lack of accountability kills. The lack of agency to articulate and exercise one's civic rights kills. Poverty kills. These are eminently political issues. These are, indeed, feminist issues. At the moment, I am thrown into the emergency of learning to deal with my grief and learning to help mother her children—the same way that Anta came with me to northern Senegal when I was conducting fieldwork and helped and supported my work, and nurtured my child as her own. I am now—with her husband, my parents, my grandmother, and my sisters—part of the army of other-parents who have stood up to continue her legacy and take care of her children. She left us the hard task of dealing with her presence-absence and the joy of bringing the collective back into the labour of love that is parenting. No doubt it will not be a peaceful and tranquil journey; it will also include difficult debates and consensus making.

More than ever, alone in the crowd with my grief, together in family, I believe in the power of collective organizing and in the power of storytelling as a way to be present to one self and to show up for others.

As Amina Mama says,

> Writing offers us the means to move beyond the crush and confusion of the immediate present. Writing also offers us the chance to maintain our sense of who we are, self-respect intact, in the knowledge that we have challenged the paradigms bestowed upon us by histories and herstories that have not been of our own making. As such it is often therapeutic as well as political, subversive as well as transformative. Above all it is an irresistible temptation. Write, rewrite, and write again. (20)

Conclusion

Raising a child is difficult, and it requires kindness to and solidarity with parents. In this chapter, I have shared how the legacy of parenting from my mother and my own realities led me to also invent another way to coparent with my husband and to build bridges with other individuals from mostly non-Western backgrounds and in the diaspora who also identify as feminist parents. Parenting is also such an important terrain that I believe it must be repoliticized because educating our children not to dominate or oppress is not only a fight against our patriarchal and capitalist societies but also a fight against the self. Parents have so much potential power in their hands that I believe there is much potential in rethinking the way we parent and the way we let also our children guide us into parenting them better by constantly negotiating our shared relationships, iteratively and endlessly talking back to them and listening to them, as well as reengineering our much fluid and nondefinitive parenting pact. Parenting my daughter and my sister's children has taught me to be kinder to my parents and to other parents and carers around me. Parenting is truly a labour of love, and the goal is for everyone to remain alive and together in the end, despite the extremely bumpy and less travelled road.

Endnotes

1. Taken from Aidoo, Ama Ata, "A Young Woman's Voice Does Not Break, It Grows Firmer."
2. The quote is taken from Warsan Shire, *Teaching My Mother How to Give Birth*. flipped eye publishing, 2011.
3. "Womanism" is a term coined by Alice Walker in *In Search of Our Mother's Gardens: Womanist Prose* to conceptualise a definition of feminism that is not based on gender equality but on race and colour. It is universalistic, and she defines a womanist as "A woman who loves another woman, sexually and/or nonsexually. She appreciates and prefers women's culture, women's emotional flexibility ... [she] is committed to the survival and wholeness of an entire people, male and female. Not a separatist, except periodically for health ... loves the spirit.... loves struggle. Loves herself. Regardless" (xi-xii).

Works Cited

Aidoo, Ama Ata. *After the Ceremonies: New and Selected Poems*. University of Nebraska Press, 2017.

Bâ, Mariama. *So Long a Letter*. Translated by Moudpe Bode-Thomas. Heinemann, 2008.

Cho, Sumi, et al. "Toward a Field of Intersectionality Studies: Theory, Applications, and Praxis." *Signs*, 2013, vol. 38, 4, pp. 786-810.

Crenshaw, Kimberlé, "Demarginalizing the Intersection of Race and Sex: A Black Feminist Critique of Antidiscrimination Doctrine, Feminist Theory and Antiracist Politics." *University of Chicago Legal Forum*, 1989, vol. 1, pp. 139-67.

Diagne, Pathé. *Pouvoir politique traditionnel en Afrique occidentale: essais sur les institutions politiques précoloniales*. Karthala. 1967.

Diop, Abdoulaye, Bara. *La Famille Wolof: tradition et changement*. Editions Karthala, 1985.

Gikandi, Simon. "A Voyage Round My Daughter." *Fathers and Daughters: An Anthology of Exploration*, edited by Ato Quayson, Ayebia Clarke, 2008, pp. 46-72.

Lorde, Audre. *Sister Outsider. The Transformation of Silence into Language and Action*. Crossing Press, 1977.

Mama, Amina. "Why We Must Write: Personal Reflections on Linking the Alchemy of Science with the Relevance of Activism." *Agenda: Empowering Women for Gender Equity*, vol. 46, 2000, pp. 13-20.

Nayyirah Waheed, Nayyirah. "Emotional Nutrition." *Herdacity*, 2020, herdacity.org/women-in-rebellion-finding-your-voice/. Accessed 23 Feb. 2020.

Oyèwùmí, Oyèrónké, *What Gender Is Motherhood: Changing Yorùbá Ideals of Power, Procreation, and Identity in the Age of Modernity*. Palgrave MacMillan, 2016.

Shire, Warsan. *Teaching My Mother How to Give Birth*. flipped eye publishing, 2011.

Walker, Alice. *In Search of Our Mothers' Gardens: Womanist Prose*. Harcourt Brace Jovanovich Publishers, 1984.

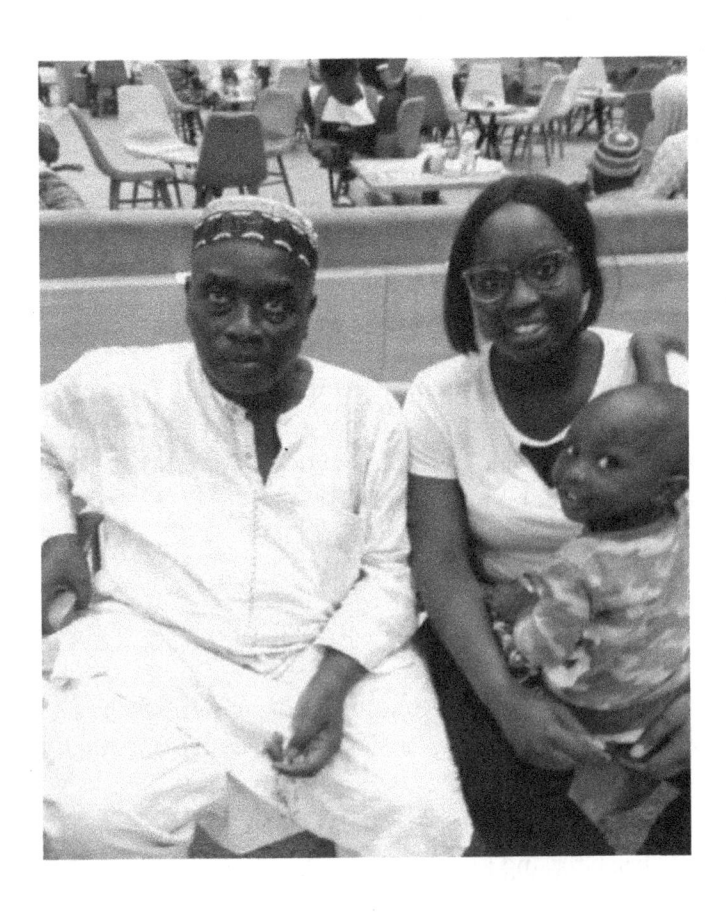

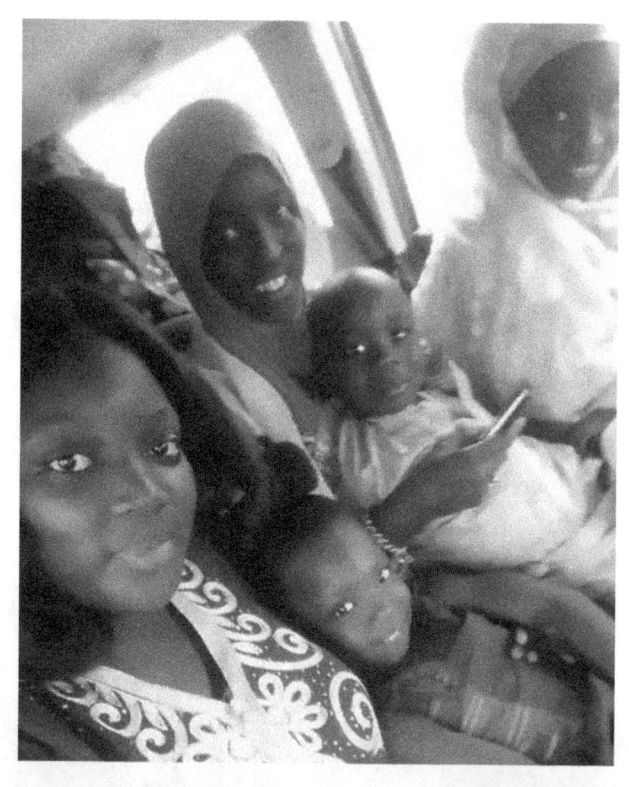

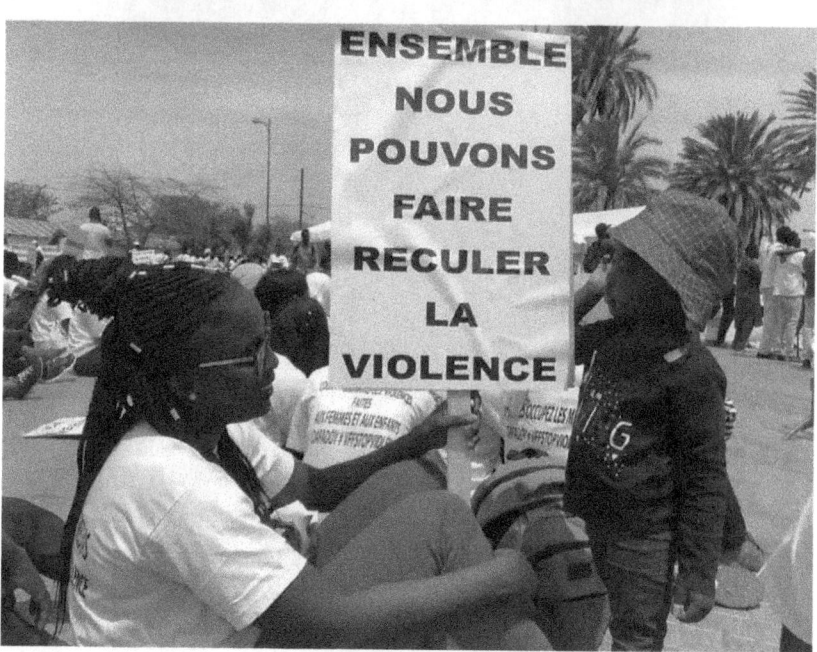

"A YOUNG WOMAN'S VOICE DOES NOT BREAK, IT GROWS FIRMER"

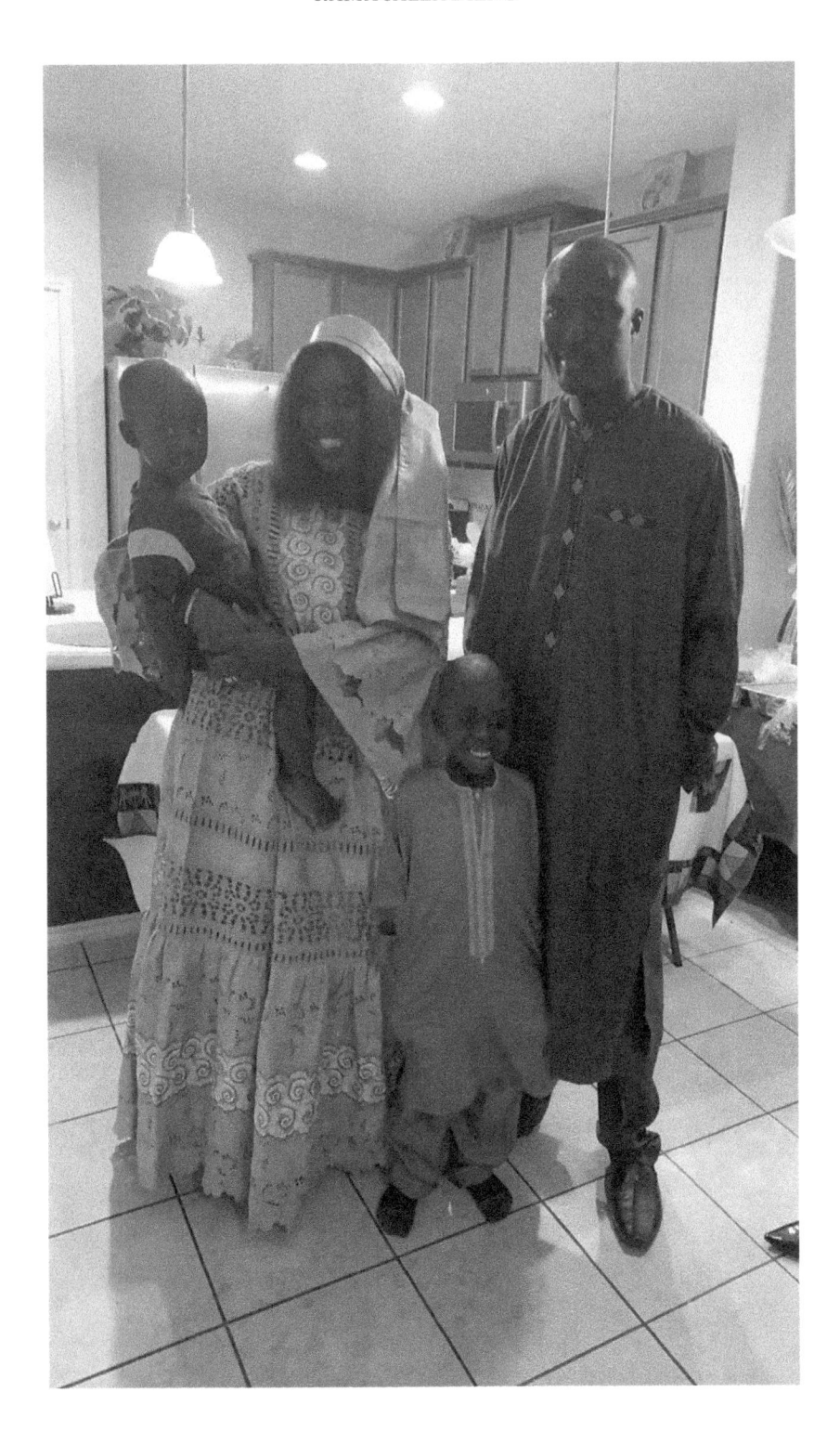

"A YOUNG WOMAN'S VOICE DOES NOT BREAK, IT GROWS FIRMER"

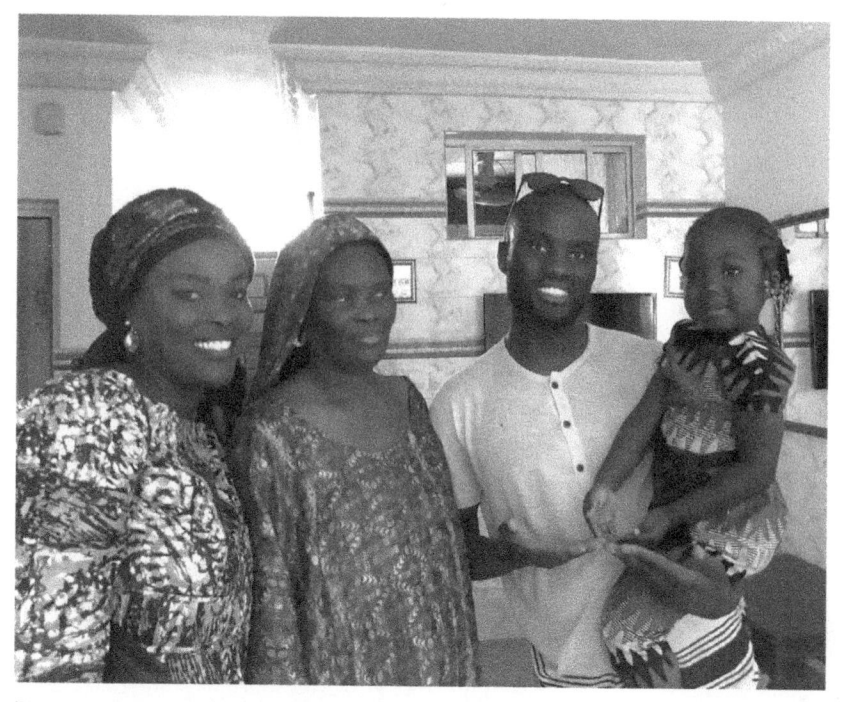

Pictures of our very large family.

Chapter 10

Feminist Parenting from the Lens of a Muslim Woman

Kula Fofana

Introduction

Patriarchy is firmly entrenched in Liberia, as it is in many countries in the world. Gender roles are ascribed based on sex. For example, women are seen as the caretakers of the home, whereas men are groomed to be providers of the home. This arrangement loosely translates to women staying home and taking care of the children and husbands, and to men working and earning resources for the family. Additionally, children are taught to obey their parents and are constantly reminded of Ephesian 6:1, of biblical text that emphasizes the obedience of children. As a predominantly Christian majority country, yet constitutionally secular, religious institutions in Liberia reinforce the teaching of these roles.

Like Christianity, Islam teaches the concept of obedience to the Creator and parents; it also ascribes roles to individuals in the society. In the spheres of worship, both men and women are held to the same standards and are expected to pursue an equal understanding of their faith. For women, they are taught to care for the home and children and are granted the right to select or divorce a husband. These roles, however, are not limited to the rearing of children, choosing a partner, and contributing to the family; they extend beyond the social realm of the home. A major challenge to women has been the policy and practices of patriarchal societies, including Islamic ones, that have oppressed women. In some instances, religious revelations have been (mis)interpreted from a cultural and traditional lens that fits the social political context of a particular regime. For example, the wearing of the veil holds a significant place for both Muslim men and women. Men and women are especially encouraged to dress modestly. Although there is no explicit Qur'anic exhortation for covering the head for Muslim women, many women choose to do so as a matter of choice (Macdonald). In Turkey in the late 1920s under the rule of Reza Shah Pahlavi, women were forcefully required to remove the veil. This was the ruler's attempt at ensuring conformity with the European concept of modernity (Mirrazavi).

In contemporary society today, the concept of choice for Muslim women is central to the practice of their faith. Amid media stereotypes of Muslim women as oppressed and in need of liberation, Muslim women are continuously reclaiming their narrative. Their decisions concerning whether or not to marry, have children, to be in a polygamous marriage, to work outside of the home, to aspire for political leadership, or to attain higher education have not only uphold the agency of Muslim women but provided them autonomy; they have used their religion as a source of empowerment, not the version portrayed deliberately by institutions of patriarchy. It is on those bases that I see my feminism as African, intersectional, Islamic, hijabi, womanist, and humanist.

In this chapter, I share my experiences from being a part of two generations of a Muslim polygamous household and how those experiences, coupled with the social, political, and economic nature of my country, have affected my understanding of feminist parenting; my intention is not to degrade the institution of polygamy but to understand it. The chapter also discusses my concept of feminism, which is African, intersectional, Islamic, hijabi, womanist, and humanist. It is important to me today to make such distinctions because often time, feminism is placed in a box that is centred on first- and second-wave of feminism, which is radical and often based on Western ideas. Because my feminism is intersectional, its conceptualization is based on one's experience and the vantage point from which they speak. I also argue even though there is no conclusive to-do list for parenting feminist, experiences from one's upbringing can have a toxic, wholesome, or somewhere in between impact on one's parenting style. The opportunity to relearn and unlearn previously held concepts of "how to" can be liberating, but, most importantly, encouraging behavior change in patriarchal societies by men (and women) is where the real revolution lies.

I grew up in Liberia, a country that has had periods of prolonged conflicts. Prior to the political upheaval in 1990, both my parents worked outside of the home. Household chores were shared among the children regardless of sex. Chores were given based on one's capability. For example, my older siblings would fetch water, cook, and clean until I was old enough to do my share. However, I would help out as I felt necessary. It wasn't required. Dad seldom chimed in. For the most part, my mother was the early bird, as she woke everyone up, including Dad, for the morning prayers and breakfast that she prepared. Our family was a nontraditional Muslim family as expected by the society in which we found ourselves. Schooling was a requirement for all, including the girls. Unlike my family, some parents, particularly in rural communities, made choices to send their boys to school and not the girls. Girls were groomed to prepare for marriage. There is a particular Liberian phrase that says "a woman's *kenja* (loosely translated as "load") cannot be left by the wayside"—meaning women are the property of the man. Every woman is expected to be picked by a man, some kind of man. There is a particular timeline that women are expected to go through: be born, grow up, join the traditional society (*sande*), get married, and have children. In traditional societies, men, too, have their timeline: be born, grow up, get educated, work hard enough, marry wives, and provide for the family. Such practices are common not only among Muslim families but all families, including Christian ones. Despite being a predominantly Christian country, customary and statutory laws operate in the same space.

African, Intersectional, Islamic, Hijabi, Womanist, and Humanist

My feminism from an African perspective values African traditions that respect both girls and boys and that seeks to protect and support women and people of society. It also respects Africans traditions that promote the diversity of the continent. Although racial inequality is important, our challenges as women on the continent are seldom racial. An intersectional feminist approach means understanding that from my particular standpoint as an African feminist, I may be privileged or disadvantaged by a particular situation. I do not claim to know or represent every situation or oppression that women of different

Role Revisal, Name Change, and the Implication for Masculinity

Liberia fought through fourteen years of civil war. Families were divided, killed, and persecuted. My family and my husband's particularly suffered persecution and oppression. Being a part of the Muslim minority, our families were a target of oppression. My father was a professor and worked in the government. His work exposed him to many people. Because of his surname, religion, and being a man, he was a target for either joining a warring faction or being killed. During the heart of the crisis and the many years we spent displaced in refugee camps, when periods of hostilities broke out, Mom became the man of the house. She left us strapped to one another while she would go looking for food under flying bullets. Dad was not going to risk his life to be in the streets. Mom did though. We did not see this as an issue, even though our society, like many others, pressures men to be the primary care person for the family.

The changing of surnames after marriage has become a controversial subject in recent years. Before colonialism, African women maintained the surnames of their fathers or the location they were from, even in a polygamous union. In Islam, for instance, many women were referred to by the surname of their fathers during the time of the Prophet (PBUH). It was revealed in the Holy Qur'an that people be called by the names of their fathers, as it pleases the Creator.

My husband's mothers maintained their families' surnames after their marriage, but my mother took my father's when it came to legal documentation. However, during the crisis, every time Dad came in close contact with rebel groups or a warring faction, he had to change his surname to that of my mother's. The Liberian war had many aspects. Ethnicity was key. Mandingoes and Muslims were particularly targeted. My mother is Vai, which is also a Muslim majority tribal group. My dad constantly changed his identity to that of my mother's for protection.

Upon marrying my husband, I chose to keep my surname, as it is an identity that I cherish and in fulfilment of my religious obligation. This is something that is frowned upon in our society. Women are pressured to change their identity to that of their husband's upon marriage.

Name changing for conviction or convenience does not seem to change in practice the person you are, and letting people make that choice for themselves is important. I would love my kids to make the choice for themselves. Whether my future sons take on their wife's name or my daughters maintain their father's name is a choice that they have to make for themselves, and it is something I would want to leave for them to decide when they are old enough.

The Decision to Have a Child before Marriage

Growing up in a religiously conscious household with stricter rules as to when and who we invite in our reproductive space was suffocating but at the same time liberating. It was liberating because we had to wait until marriage to have children with the right person, which gave us more time to focus on other aspects of our lives, including education. It was suffocating because we could not understand why we were held to different standards than those of our relatives or our parents. Before Dad and Mom married, they had kids in their previous relationships. We were probably being prevented from committing the sins of our neighbors, families, or parents, since having kids before marriage was and is still considered a sin. As this is seriously frowned upon, many kids resort to having an illegal abortion. Families pay little attention to reproductive education for their children. That marriage is over romanticized and overrated is something ostensibly perplexing.

I questioned my parents, mostly my mom, on many things that I considered confusing. Many years ago, I remember asking my mom why she always gave my brothers and dad so much more meat than me when she cooked. She said when I grew up, I would understand. I felt that was her way of practicing inequality, so I devised a strategy. When my brothers and dad were not around, I would take portion of their meat and add it to mine in protest of the unequal treatment. Of course, I would be reprimanded again and again.

Having a child for me was something I had planned out. Married or not, I had to be in a place where I was able to cater for my child, but it was not going to stand in the way of my career—a struggle many women, including my friends, go through. Having a family or children should not compromise your career but complement it. It is a difficult decision to decide between family and career for fear of losing one to the other.

I met my now husband a year before graduation. Letting someone for the first time into my personal and reproductive space involved a lot of learning and unlearning. We had Iman, our beautiful cutie, after three years of dating and married three years later. We were not going to let the pressure of our families and friends dictate the course of our relationship.

Feminist Parenting and the Way We See It

I have been a feminist for as long as I can remember. Having a strong woman—my mother—in my life has been a blessing, as she has helped me see the world as larger than what society, tradition, and custom taught me. My husband sees himself as a feminist ally and says so publicly because he believes women can better understand how patriarchal structures continue to hold them back. As a man, he can help by publically supporting initiatives that are geared to helping women and girls; he himself personally funds scholarship initiatives for girls. In male-only spaces, he makes his thoughts on women or feminism known.

Feminist parenting takes a lot of learning and unlearning for both of us. My concept of feminist mothering is seeing motherhood from a broad spectrum. By this, I mean incorporating feminist ideals in my everyday parenting, which can include correcting sexist language in everyday conversations, choosing outfits, toys, or other items for Iman, her male and female cousins, and ensuring that our oldest son learns to cook so that he doesn't assume cooking is a craft only for women. It also means communicating that the role each individual brings to the table is not determined by their sex. For example, my husband can decide to prepare breakfast, lunch, and dinner while I do the laundry, and that does not make him any less of a man or me any more of a woman. Everyone should contribute in an equal way. Times are different, and helping our children navigate with us through life is never easy. Both of our upbringings were slightly different, but for our family of five, we build our understanding on the power of communication, boundaries, choices, and language; we see them as key to our family's value.

Communication is important for our family. The power to listen, be heard, feel heard, and be able to express ourselves without being judged is something we constantly value. This includes between us as parents and for all of the kids in our clan, whether biological or adopted. Communication doesn't have to always be about good grades and expectations. Sometimes it is about their best friends, favorite memories, or deeper issues. Boundaries are also paramount for us. We grew up in a society in which the parent-children relationship was like rulers and the ruled. Sometimes we are tempted to switch to that mode but quickly remind ourselves that we are all human and need a collective approach to the parent-children relationship. We are learning to keep healthy boundaries with our children and our individual selves. We are constantly learning to recognize the other beings in our family and that they too exist and their voices and privacy need be respected. But we do this without giving up our agency as parents.

Choice is a concept that has broadened our family values. Respecting the choice of our kids while differentiating what is a healthy or an unhealthy choice is a struggle we have. Sometimes it takes a lot of negotiating. For instance, sometimes it is a choice between wants and needs, what they can live with or without. Most times, it is a win-lose scenario.

Language and being open minded are also important to us, as is the understanding that people are different and everyone deserves respect, regardless of who they are, where they are from, or what they look like. We teach our kids that being a boy or a girl does not define what a person can and cannot do. We try to decolorize our minds concerning pink vs blue, Barbie doll vs Lego toys, and many others, which has been a tall order especially with influences from friends, families, school, and the media. For our family of five—that is our adopted daughter, Iman, her brother, and my husband and me—it can be a handful sometimes, but we are learning as we progress. We are hopeful yet very far from perfect. Sometimes our policy and practice are in competition with each other, but we are not giving up.

Iman is already in a league of her own in that she has already begun questioning what she thinks is wrong or right, despite being so young. She tells her dad to speak a certain way when he seems angry. For example, when she turned two, a friend got her a Barbie doll and another bought her a set of Lego blocks. She swore she would not take the doll and didn't want to have anything to do with it, but she sprinted to get the Lego blocks and then started constructing.

Parenting from Afar

My quest for education and to contribute to the world around me takes me away from home a lot. Balancing my career, family, and work is difficult and comes with a price. Missing out on some amazing milestones and conversations especially for Iman, who is the young one, is tough. I tried to make the best out of the physical time we have together when we can. Keeping in touch as much as I can and making up for lost time helps a lot—thanks to technology. My husband is the strong one here. This is the longest I have been away from home, and the struggle is real. I studied in London for a period of two years. He works in Doha, Qatar. We also have an active home in Liberia. Long distance relationships are hard, and a commitment from both partners to step up is very important. This is the toughest test for our relationship. Our commitment to making it work takes plenty of sacrificing and being considerate. Making sure the other partner stays up to date with what's going on with the family, including the children, is essential, but it is hard to keep up to date on an hour-to-hour basis. It is okay to miss out on some. Not always feeling guilty and forgiving yourself are key. As career-driven mothers, it is instinctive to sometimes feel that we are not giving our best selves to the family; however, sometimes, the men in our lives do not feel as guilty as we do when the table turns. It is important to see the bigger picture. As much as we may want to instill feminist values in our children, there is no perfect way to do it. You learn, unlearn, and relearn as you navigate along. It may turn out that your kids may or may not be feminists.

Conclusion

Although there is no specific way to be a feminist parent, my experience growing up in a polygamous household with many siblings and seeing that my parents did not give any child preferential treatment and disciplined everyone equally made me realize that individuals can decide for themselves what to incorporate in their family values despite what society tells them. As a Muslim couple, we are constantly committed to working with our kids to make it work. My feminism is African, intersectional, Islamic, hijabi, womanist, and humanist.

Works Cited

Macdonald, Myra. "Muslim Women and the Veil." *Feminist Media Studies*, vol. 6, no. 1, 2006, pp. 7-23.

Mirrazevi, Firouzeh. "The Removing of Hijab in Iran." *Iran Review*, 2020, www.iranreview.org/content/Documents/The-Removing-of-Hijab-in-Iran.htm. Accessed 19 Feb. 2020.

Part II

Parenting Is Political: Of Feminist Mothers' Struggles and Resistance

Chapter 11

The Necessity of Rage and the Politics of Feminist Parenting

Masana Ndinga-Kanga

"Mother is the name for God in the lips and hearts of little children."
—William Makepeace Thackeray, *Vanity Fair*, 184

Introduction

I come from a strong matriarchal family, which at first glance may seem unusual for a patriarchal society like that found in South Africa. Some of the presence of matriarchs in my mother's line was by design—a consequence of the intentional political landscape of the country. Most of the presence of strong matriarchs was by a series of unfortunate events. The nature of apartheid South Africa often removed black men from a primary parenting role because of the migrant labour system. My maternal grandfather was one such man who, because of the needs of his eight offspring, travelled to Johannesburg to work as a security guard while my mother and her siblings remained in the village engaged in smallholder farming under the strict, watchful eye of my grandmother. The burden of raising so many young children meant that she was often heavy handed; her children often lamented in their adult years how her use of force was a mechanism of control that hurt them in different ways. When my grandfather passed, my mother assumed the role of matriarch—having been one of the few women to leave the village, study medicine, and, consequently, put her siblings, their children, and her own through school.

I saw in both my grandmother and mother the embodiment of sacrifice that left me tense at the ways in which parenting seemed to strip women of the capacity to act in their own self-interest, even if it resulted in familial wellbeing. I observed the ways in which these women with great wit, force, and determination carved out options for economic mobility for their children—making choices that often chipped away at their own peace. In those times, during the early nineties, my parents religiously took us to church every Sunday morning. The old, white Anglican bishop would take us through Eucharist each Easter, reminding us of the great love and sacrifice of the Father. Despite these teachings, I could not relate to a patriarchal figure of redemption; I saw true sacrifice and love in the women that had laid the path before me. Yet I felt great pain at the cost of this sacrifice for these women, who sometimes bit their tongues so that one day I could speak.

In navigating these tensions, I argue in this chapter that feminist parenting is fundamentally political and that rage is a core component of claiming a life where self-sacrifice is not the default disposition that young black girls are inducted into through observing their mothers. Rather than look to Judeo-Christian templates of parenting, which serve to placate the necessary rage at class, sex and race oppression, feminist parents must create their own nodes of coherence. Rage at injustice can serve as the initial catalyst into autonomy and self-care—essential principles of feminism that are often subverted through framing rage by black women under the stereotype of the angry black woman. This chapter begins with an exploration of my own background to understanding rage as critical for feminist parenting. It then reflects on the problematic assumptions belying Judeo-Christian frameworks for rage and parenting, before turning to the political impetus behind feminist parenting. This chapter then demonstrates how I have sought to embody new ways of parenting for my child, before concluding with my lessons and hopes given this new framing. I argue that legitimating anger is critical to reclaiming its important role in liberation across social, economic, and political spheres, not just for the mother as an individual in her interpersonal life but also as a political actor in a violently patriarchal society.

Background—My Induction into Motherhood

Despite being a maternal and nurturing person, I approached motherhood with skepticism. I feared the wilting away of myself in the name of self-sacrificial parenting. I knew that to fall into that pattern would be to kick dust into the weary eyes of the matriarchs before me. I had also entered marriage with some theoretical knowledge of the workings of feminism in an egalitarian heterosexual relationship but did not realize how little I truthfully practiced it for myself. I was quickly disgruntled at the inequality of my emotional labour that also uniquely intersected with bearing the financial burden in the home. When we married, I thought that we had the necessary groundwork to make the commitment last: we both had a feminist ethos (his more coherent than mine), a shared faith that we engaged with skepticism, and a commitment to check ourselves. Yet I found that there were far more insidious patriarchal dynamics that we both upheld—over and above our individual traumas. Furthermore, the currency of my faith rapidly devalued in the context of the self-sacrificial narrative that informed my previous commitment to Christianity. I rapidly found myself at odds with a Christian dogma of women's submission and compliance, codified through weekly teachings that I had no time for while trying to keep myself, our home, and our child afloat. I fell quickly into the restrictive framework laid before me. I had hoped for a more utopian outworking of feminism that held and nurtured both me and my then partner and our soon to be child.

I stepped into motherhood disillusioned with marriage and my own functioning as a political being in an intimate space, desperate for mutual respect. Giving birth suddenly placed a responsibility on my shoulders to embody a feminism that was clear cut and easy. My daughter needed to see me practice this every day, I thought with conviction. My own process to get to this place was awkward and complex. Rather than articulate my feminism in research and intellectual debates (as had been the case up until that point), I noted with urgency in the days before my child was born that I needed outwork my feminism. I recalled that my child needed to see options of parenting that did not require women to sacrifice themselves to the point of poor mental health and exhaustion, especially in a context where I had the socioeconomic resources to demonstrate this—a privilege my own trauma would not let me tap into. From the day she was born, Elikia (now four years old) was wide eyed and observant; she watched and mimicked me so closely that by two, I realized that I was teaching her how to be a black woman through my behaviour. The stakes were too high. I did not want her to learn from me how to wilt away. I wanted to try an alternative way of being, which broadened my shoulders to carry the weight of the wrestle for justice and equality for my daughter, but I also presented her with the option to choose herself and her wellbeing as part of the revolutionary process.

Rather than maintain the comfort of others in the face of patriarchal oppression, it was important to teach Elikia that she had the power and agency to give voice to her frustration and use that to move herself to a place of wellbeing. I wish I had the capacity to articulate then what I have since learned to grasp in my own experience of motherhood—that feminist parenting as a black woman is fundamentally political in both intimate and social spheres and that legitimating rage (of the black feminine) is the central mechanism through which I can pass on tools of being in the world to my daughter.

Resisting the Theological Template for Parenting

Religion has played a complex role in the personal, communal, and societal spheres of African society, and Christianity is no exception. Since its inception in the continent, it has been part of an oppressive power structure, contributed to internalized inferiority complexes of predominantly black peoples, and supported submission to colonial powers. For example, in South Africa, apartheid philosophy was borne out of Calvinist theology. Religion has also presented modes of being within the more intimate confines of the family and has clearly articulated a patriarchal power structure that further emphasized submission: of child and woman to father and husband, and if through race: of black people to the white man and woman. This double jeopardy organized itself along gender, class, and race hierarchies that ultimately worked in unison to disenfranchise black women and their children, not only to black men but also to white power. Although the latter has in principle been dismantled (but not in practice), it is only in recent decades that the insidious patriarchal nature of Christian philosophy has been exposed for its damaging effects on intimate relationships within the black intimate space. Within the confines of this doctrine, the feminine is hidden as the parenting relationship between God and His children is framed as masculine—the Father being the epitome of love, despite His insatiable thirst for blood and sacrifice. It is important to ask why this love cannot be mutually beneficial and require not only sacrifice and compromise but also mutual respect.

Despite the framing of the ultimate love by deity as masculine, the practicalities of parenting have historically fallen to women as the primary custodians of rearing future generations. It was only when I left the confines of this religious paradigm of race, class, and sex power dynamics that I learned that to parent a young black girl child required a profound and spiritual respect for rage, happiness, and autonomy. Rather than look to a patriarchal configuration of redemption, becoming a mother forced me to embody for myself rage, happiness, and autonomy as a first step towards our mutual liberation. I have not raised my daughter to idolize self-sacrifice as the ultimate expression of love. Rather, autonomy and shared care become critical, practical expressions of love. However, when these dynamics are violated, rage at injustice is a legitimate outcome. It is only within giving voice to anger that I then began to embark on a parental journey that sat comfortably in defiance of racist, sexist, and classist readings of motherhood within the South African political economy. I found that this was the only way I could sustainably be a black mother to a black girl child in a world that was primarily against these characteristics over which she would have no design. A faith-based approach to parenting did not create a radical space for me to do this.

In a country where most people identify as Christian and use that ideology to shape their parental approach, it is important to understand the intersection of family, identity, and politics in moulding a feminist theory of parenting for young, black female parents like myself. A new form of feminist parenting, beyond that articulated in Judeo-Christianity, thus has to recognize race, class and sex to be truthful to its claims of liberation and salvation – claiming the feminine as essential for freedom within, and externally, in a world that is still finding a praxis for feminist parenting.

Parenting as Political

Winnie Madikizela-Mandela once reflected on the intimate link between being a black single mother and the political climate of apartheid South Africa. With Nelson Mandela imprisoned for five decades, she observed that her experience of motherhood was fundamentally political in part because of how she was forced into resistance against a state that stood against everything she was: black, woman, mother to black children, and defiant. Her political experience of parenting was also the result of the havoc wreaked on black families by structural oppression, including the impact of migrant labour on the family nucleus. In order to meet their economic gains, apartheid society required the movement of black bodies from the hinterland to the centre to supply cheap labour. Families disintegrated under the pressure to meet livelihoods as black men travelled to mines, urban areas, or farms and left behind families of mothers and children—or more often grandmothers and children, as black women often travelled as well to serve as domestic workers for predominantly white women.

The nebulous family unit was further complicated by a mode of parenting that consisted of internalized racist and sexist patterns, where children were taught to self-preserve, to stay on the right side of the law, to behave appropriately, and to not antagonize structures of white supremacy that were contained and sustained by white people for their privilege and by black people for their safety. Making oneself small and shrinking one's existence were paralleled by broader societal structures of self-preservation in the face of threats to safety. Key examples included nonviolent movements or practicing obedience to parental, elderly, or church moralities as well as other structures. The disappearance of voice and the internalization of inferiority became insidious mechanisms of containing righteous anger, the legitimacy of happiness, and the right to personal autonomy.

For young females, their self-actualization was further limited within the structures of patriarchy and violent masculinity that characterized apartheid society—an experience of gendered violence that continues to feature prominently today in South Africa, where one in five women are subject to sexual violence in their lifetimes. And, thus, through generations, learned behaviours are passed down to children and are informed by race, class, and gender within a political economy that benefits from the oppression of the young black female child. The process of unlearning also takes generations, even in matriarchal families like my own. Despite there being a significant number of female-headed households in my family, I found slow iterations of feminism being handed down. My grandmother's mistrust of men because of the ways in which they (physically and emotionally) left women to rear children translated into my own mother's desire for more out of life than just marriage. My mother, reared in the rural areas of northern South Africa, subsequently went on to obtain a doctorate and an MBA; she also qualified as a medical doctor despite being the first in her family to graduate. She gave her three daughters, me included, a way of being that prioritized practical feminism, although she did not use the language for it. She lived it. Yet the more insidious patterns of patriarchy within the home were more difficult to shake through the generations, and the burden of care overwhelmingly fell to these women even when they were within the social safety of marriage—it did not translate into mutual respect. Learning to be different in the intimate space was a lesson I needed to learn for myself.

Through decades of social engineering, single mothers have come to head many homes in South Africa, yet the articulation of a feminist identity for single mothers is not one formally handed down through the family lineage of learning. Feminist ideals could be transferred through informal ways of being and through formal and informal education in schools, public campaigns, and social media. The informal is of most interest. In my own experience as a granddaughter, daughter, and mother, there have been processes of a strengthened feminist identity that have become more coherent, as I have sought to wrestle with the world my child may one day inherit. My grandmother refused to speak English and Afrikaans, thus harnessing the power of xiTsonga as a legitimate tool of expression with her children and grandchildren. This political resistance, while small scale, challenged the expansion of coloniality in South Africa at the time and has continued to disrupt spaces of Eurocentrism in the postapartheid era and in our home. An extension of this type of personalized political resistance also includes my mother's refusal to attend her graduation in defiance of the racist higher education system, where, despite all odds, she graduated in medicine in the 1980s at the height of resistance against apartheid. In both these instances (and many other undocumented), my mother and grandmother used their bodies as sites of resistance in ways that challenged the mundanity of violence enforced on black women's bodies—policing the ways of being, speaking, or learning. Each generation has developed nuances of feminist articulation more highly attuned to the complex interaction of sex and power in its context. This indirect transfer of feminist power has supported my direct transfer of a political feminism to my daughter, where I clearly speak to her about political resistance as essential to her own ability to exercise her agency. Articulating anger is a core component of this learning. In my mother and grandmother, I saw a self-sacrifice and well-regulated rage that ultimately cost them rest, where the politics of appropriateness for black women wears them down at work and home. I have been privileged to see my mother embody anger in my lifetime. Because of the tediousness of politeness, I wish this was something that she had expressed and legitimated sooner. But the lesson came, and for me, it has been an instrumental tool of my own feminist articulation. I could only learn this tool by watching her practice it. She was the best feminist teacher to give rise to my self-actualization.

Rage and anger are critical, especially where passiveness and submission have been internalized and where negative stereotypes of angry black woman abound in popular discourse. By enacting anger and demonstrating its utility, black feminist parents can show how harmful self-sacrificial obligations are to the realization of wellbeing for black women and girls. Resisting the power structures that enforce a style of parenting that requires the proverbial (and often literal) blood of the mother is crucial for a world that seeks to protect women and girl children. They must have autonomy and the right to self-autonomy. At times, aspiring to this dynamic may seem idealistic and far removed from structural inequality. However, I argue that situating them within the political economy—and thus making parenting political—is fundamental to the reading of parental responsibilities as part of a broader commitment to class, race, and gender justice. The pursuit of happiness, for example, must be read as more than the desire for middle-class luxuries; instead, happiness must result from the pursuit of autonomy resulting from a keen awareness of the injustices of the world (and even the home) and the capacity to move and create change. Taken together, tools have helped me articulate a way of being in relation to my child that gives her (emotional, social, and political) space in a context where that is ill afforded to black girl children. I hope that this thinking can be the floor to her ceiling in whatever path she chooses, and more so that this path would be one that continues the realization of equity for black girl children.

On the Importance of Rage

> "We can disagree and still love each other unless your disagreement is rooted in my oppression and denial of my humanity and right to exist."
> —Robert Jones Jr., qtd. in *Son of Baldwin*

I learned too late that rage was a necessary response in life, not only for its quality but also for its impact on my survival. Despite the church narratives of righteous anger captured by Jesus throwing up the tables of those selling goods in his father's house, rage remained elusive to me because it was validated by the morality of Christian righteousness. This complex relationship with rage was also situated within not only the negative discourse of black anger in broader society but also the stereotypical framing of angry black women, which has often been used to delegitimize the healthy response to experiences of violation.

Despite public displays of anger at racial injustice gaining legitimacy through the student movements in South Africa, queer black women were met with violence after their demonstration against patriarchal power structures of the #FeesMustFall. Increasingly, women emboldened by their frustration at the student movement have called for the struggle for decolonization to include an outright rejection of patriarchy and its damaging influence on the public and private spheres of noncisgender, nonheterosexual peoples. The anger of these young black women represented the legitimization of rage in the face of systemic violation—in that moment articulated in public. I internalized these processes to give voice to my own rage. At the time that the protests were happening, I worked at the University of Cape Town and had experienced being the only black female researcher on staff and being asked to clean a senior white male's office. That year, I was also pregnant and deeply frustrated at the ways in which racist patriarchy undermined my capacity to participate as an equal in the work place but also as a soon-to-be-mother. What determined whose rage was legitimate? How could I know that my rage was legitimate? I needed to make legitimate my feelings of injustice and use my rage to move.

Night after night, I would ruminate on my anger. Sometimes my anger was about the big things: the killing of people of colour across the world, the impact of colonization, the rape of women and children, and many other societal ills. Often, my anger was about my experience of these things—the experience of multiple rapes as a child, seeing my well-educated mother shrink within her home under the weight of patriarchal expectations, or the ways in which homes were empty of men, even when they were physically present. The daily experiences of discrimination and the subtler experiences of patriarchy chipped away at my sense of self until the voice of the world became the voice with which I used to talk to myself. Feminism became my lifeline because it is the political, social, economic, and intimate process by which I can be an entire human being, articulate my aspirations, and have these realized in ways that are equitable and just rather than dehumanizing and exploiting. Feminism is the process by which I have learned to legitimate myself and the many women within me, including those before and those to come. By extension, feminist parenting requires that I pass on the modes of legitimization to my daughter while actively taking steps daily to parent differently.

Practically, this has meant speaking differently to Elikia, hearing her even in the early days when her sentences were indecipherable. I try to show Elikia what it is to be heard; I stop often to acknowledge her conversationally rather than primarily through instruction. Her first full sentence was "I don't like that," in which she communicated to me her agency and I respected her autonomy to dislike things that I do. Sometimes the things she communicates are small; for example, she does not like packing away her toys or taking medicine. I acknowledge these and try to explain to her why it is important to take a multivitamin. Other times, she communicates big things that she does not like—hugging or kissing people known and unknown, having a big afro that looks cute but is very painful to comb, or even being fun when she is tired. I have to stop myself in these moments and actively say, as I do for some of the small things, "I understand, and it is okay for you not to do this if you do not want to." Often, I also have to demonstrate to her how to be true to how she is feeling as an option of many when she feels uncomfortable, violated, or subtly coerced. This sometimes means saying no, saying "I need time alone," or walking away from hurtful situations. Most importantly, this means moving in mind, spirit and body towards alignment of self—this part is more difficult. I am a work in progress, failing forward, as I learn what my own alignment is and how best to nurture and support that of my daughter.

THE NECESSITY OF RAGE AND THE POLITICS OF FEMINIST PARENTING

Within my parenting role, I realized that I need an internal legitimization of my own anger. I believe the political, the economic, and the structural to be intimately linked to the personal—crises of patriarchy are not just about the external world. They were also about my family, my community, my country, my continent, my people, and me. To raise my daughter with the tools to challenge structural injustice, I had to embody this process. Watching my daughter grow in this context, I saw value in what can so easily be dismissed as toddler tantrums. In moments that she did not want to engage with someone, she would say no, and when she felt upset at the dynamics (albeit related to toys or the lack of desire to eat vegetables or put on shoes) she would voice her frustration. Rather than dismiss this behaviour as delinquent, I have had to shift my own relationship to anger and acknowledge the value of her enacting her discontentment. Rather than frown upon her rage, I have had to turn to her and explicitly acknowledge that I know she is upset and explore with her the ways in which she can channel that anger into actions that edify or move her. These are the foundations of consent and bodily integrity, of standing up to imposter syndrome, or the functioning of inequality in intimate partner relationships. Doing this for her has also meant learning to do it for myself.

I have found that the problem of anger in parenting is not just that you are raising an angry black person—a threat to structures of control—but also an angry black woman who then becomes a threat to the functions of patriarchy in the home. I saw this scenario play out while living within the confines of frustration at race and gender relations in South Africa, where women are celebrated for their bold alignment with the struggle against everyday racism but shunned for their deep criticism of everyday patriarchy in the home. Thus, the other challenge of feminist parenting becomes a political wrestle within the confines of domestic life, which highlights the demand for equality in the home as it is called for in society.

Within my home, it has required an honest examination of how I respond to the frustrations of my child; I try to acknowledge her frustration before seeking to make judgment on its value. It has also required me voicing my anger and using that to move myself towards action as well as challenging my own instinctive response to shrink in the face of threats. I have seen moments of this type of being by female parents within my own life. One family member, after being hit in the face by her husband, took a picture of the effects—framing her face and displaying it in the passages of the house as a reminder of what happened and the brutality of male violence. Her anger was necessarily commemorated by herself, a template I drew on to inform my own resistance against unhealthy family dynamics.

Rather than instinctively fall into the roles required in my hetero relationship, since my daughter was born, I have been forced into self-examination, particularly because I did not want her to learn through me the functions of a small woman in a relationship. It was not until 2017 that I was able to give voice to my rage and step outside of the limitations of my own enforcement of patriarchal hetero relationships—I was faced with a mental health breakdown, and I was completely burned out, unhappy, and unable to cope with the expectations of cis-hetero relating and parenting. Thus, my process of alignment was that I would allow myself to be angry when I was angry and to voice this frustration; and to step away from situations where I was not respected out of respect of myself. The function of my anger in parenting has helped me move and occupy social and political space. I recall instances when she was an infant where white women would invade my personal space to touch my child's hair. Without consent, these women literally peeled back the baby wrap that pinned her to my body; they would expose the sleeping child on my breast to coo at how lovely she was, and I would recoil and shrink, unable to give voice to my experience of violation. This had happened on two separate occasions before I could no longer contain my rage. I angrily pointed out to the third stranger that attempted such that she had no right to expose me or to touch me or my child, and I told her that had I done the same to her, as a black woman, she would have had none of it. In that moment, my child was defenceless against the white gaze, and I would not be afforded the luxury of occupying value in a public space that was built on racist foundations. I had to use my rage to move my child to safety and, more importantly, to demonstrate to her that what might be her own experiences of injustice would require anger to move her to safety.

In the intimate space, giving legitimacy to my rage has also meant requesting separation in marriage on the premises of requiring mutual respect. I wish I had initiated the separation purely out of my own recognition of self-value. Rather, having grown up in a context where I watched the strongest woman I know bend into an origami of self-alienation, I left because I saw my daughter's big eyes take in the ways I shrunk in that love. I was inadvertently teaching her how to experience intimate partner relationships through not only my continued responsibility for the wellbeing (financial, emotional, and otherwise) of the household but also the disappearance of myself. What I assumed was the self-sacrificial nature of love, marriage and parenting ultimately did a disservice to myself to the extent that I was on the verge of a breakdown.

No matter how much I preached self-care and self-love to her, it would be the lessons of my actions that would ultimately serve as her template for being in the world—as was the case for me, learning the 'unwritten feminisms' of the matriarchs in my family. When I think back to that time, doubt still creeps over me because although some choose to stay for their children, I left for mine, and, in that, I found that I needed to leave for myself. It was my anger at the ways in which my own history was repeating itself—the rage at my own feelings of entrapment where I felt unheard—that ultimately had me move physically, spiritually, and emotionally.

Conclusion

I now contend with how parenting has forced me to practice feminism more than merely speak it. In order for my daughter to begin to articulate and embody her own freedom, she must practice it—and this is the time for learning. I learn about feminist parenting through learning about (and parenting) myself and the things that make me uncomfortable. My own internal trusting has served as the biggest cue for me to act differently, as I look within for validation of my parental, social, political, and economic decisions rather than externalize the validation of these to others. I hope that one day Elikia will do this more instinctively from the onset so that she is able to decide for herself which ways of being in the world serve her truth. I hope that this truth is committed to justice and equality. I also recognize the limitations of using anger as a mechanism to realize a feminist agenda for society, particularly because of its own emotional burden. However, I see contempt and rage as healthy human responses to injustice that have been systemically used to undermine black women to limit their capacity to mobilize and move their bodies to places of health and nurturing. I view this as a skill I learned too late to embody, but am when he opened the oven's door and were immediately dosed out. Thinking about the potential disaster that had been averted, I started crying. He checked the wiring, the sockets, the plugs, and finally examined the cookies I was baking. Obviously, before we threw them out, there was that photo he took that he will forever threaten to put up on Instagram.

It was a sad end to an effort I had made as a big gesture; I had not ventured to cook anything myself for at least a year, and homemade cookies were supposed to be my big thank you for the support he had given to me throughout my pregnancy.

*

The charcoal cookie episode, as we came to call it, is simply recounted here as a (humiliating) example of my expertise in the most traditional of wifely roles. Unlike me, my husband calls cooking a matter of common sense. He also has a perfect eye for interior décor, and all the houses that we have lived in over the last ten years have been picture perfect thanks to his interest and hard work. Although my cupboard is a hodgepodge of wrinkly clothes, his is colour coded and annoyingly perfect.

Yes, I am far from the perfect wife that South Asian moms so lovingly try to find for their sons—a demure, submissive domestic goddess, whose beauty and expertise in the kitchen fill the house with joy. Despite my feminism, the continuous digression from the traditional wifely role gives me a terrible feeling of guilt, which is only compounded when I do make an effort to be more homely and miserably fail.

I have failed at becoming a woman that society approves of in more ways than one. My stubborn denial to engage in any conversation about my reproductive choices in a society where it is common for women to be asked about "good news" the day after they get married has been a constant source of contention between me and my extended family for most of my married life.

It was only after we had already celebrated our seventh marriage anniversary that we reluctantly decided to try for a baby. Being childless seven years postmarriage and a couple of years past thirty isn't usually a conscious choice for the majority of my peers. In our seven years of marriage, my husband and I had sometimes wondered and debated the level of our readiness for a child. But there wasn't a single moment where this discussion was actually accompanied by a sense of missing a vital part of life. The lack of my own emotional engagement with the idea of motherhood often opened me up to criticism; friends and colleagues eagerly embracing their roles as mothers kept asking the same thing: "What kind of a woman doesn't want to be a mother?" The idea of motherhood as the ultimate goal and purpose of women is rooted in both cultural and religious norms. Within the Pakistani culture, the woman is seen and raised to be a child bearer, a home maker—even in educated families, girls as young as seven are pressured to learn to make *gol roties*, a flatbread that has to be rolled out in perfect rounds and made fresh for the men in the family at each meal. *Maa kay hath ki roti* (i.e., flatbreads made by the mother) are consistently portrayed as an almost sacred object within the local literature and popular media. Religion takes the value of motherhood up another notch. Ask any practicing Muslim about the status of woman in Islam, and the majority of them would come back with a single phrase—Paradise is beneath the feet of a mother. This isn't a metaphorical reference to paradise but actually refers to the paradise promised to the pious in afterlife. With motherhood, thus, connected to the ultimate reward being sought by Muslims, it is no wonder that a woman's life is seen as worthwhile only if it revolves around her identity and worth as a mother. Within this context, my own inability to feel motherly made me an anomaly of sorts—someone who did not fit into the public imagination of a good woman.

So after years of hearing covert and overt comments on this apparent flaw in my character, when we did decide to try for a child, I continued to be haunted by doubts about my ability to be an adequate mother. When the pregnancy finally happened, it was accompanied by a hundred different anxieties—would I be able to be *motherly* enough (whatever that means)? Would I be able to do justice to both the baby and my work? Would I turn bitter and resentful? Would the baby suffer from our routine?

And then the pregnancy ended in a traumatic miscarriage. It was my first trimester, and I was travelling for work. Although my doctors had given me a go ahead, my peers shook their heads in disbelief and disgust, criticizing me for prioritizing work over the baby. The first indication of trouble came before I landed at my destination. I googled the nearest hospital when I landed and was soon introduced to the term "missed miscarriage." The doctor assured me it had nothing to do with the air travel. Yet as I bled alone over the white tiles of a random hotel room, body convulsing with pain, the only thing I could think of was the fact that I had travelled against the conventional wisdom. Had my decision to fly been fatal to my child? Or was it the original choice to delay motherhood well over the prescribed age?

Given the circumstances, I was not surprised when over the next year various people told me that the miscarriage was my own fault. Whereas people had merely hinted at my lack of maternal feeling, the miscarriage seemed to trigger an aggression of sorts. I was not just childless by choice; I was someone who had deliberately endangered and killed a baby. The advice to pray for redemption and a child became common.

To me, the prayer also signifies one of the key elements defining motherhood in Pakistan. One is supposed to pray for a child, preferably male. Ask a health-related question to online mothers groups, and you'll be advised to read *wazifas*—specific combinations of Qur'anic verses that are famed to do many things for expectant mothers, from ensuring the birth of a male child to ensuring an easy, natural delivery. Questions about behavioural or health issues with children bring along another set of *wazifas*. And questions by women struggling to conceive are met with advice to pray for forgiveness for their sins. So nine years after getting married, when I conceived again, I was still shaken by doubts about my potential to actually mother. My mind went into a defensive overdrive. The amount of work that goes into running and sustaining your own organization—I would manage. My husband and I work together after all. The crazy routine with sleep deprivation—we would manage. We do stay awake half the night watching movies or reading in any case.

But even then I knew that the questions I allowed myself to be haunted by were merely logistical. The real questions were too tough to face. There is nothing like impending motherhood that makes you question your own identity. Who was I? Before feeling the kicks in my belly, I had defaulted to seeing myself as an extension of my profession. I was a journalist, a media rights activist first and foremost. I was an independent woman, financially able, professionally on par with my husband, known in the community, and reasonably successful. Yet the day the baby started kicking, my sense of self was threatened.

I had always been one of the women who initiated heated discussions about the role of men in families and wondered out aloud why women would continue to bear the brunt of childrearing. I had consoled and counselled friends who were conflicted about having children simply because they knew their career would take a hit. I understood those fears—I shared them.

Or should I say, I shared them once?

From the day I first felt the baby kicking, I felt a physical shift in my own priorities. The thoughts that came to me were sudden and unexpected. What was I doing prioritizing work over everything else? Why was my identity so ingrained in what I did? Who would I be as a mother? And, of course, would I be a good mother? What shook me most wasn't my doubt in my own ability to be a good mother; rather, it was the realization that I, someone who had always found motherhood overrated, was suddenly overwhelmed by this deep desire to do right by an unborn child.

This wasn't the me I knew.

This wasn't the me I was expecting to become.

*

The reason for this brewing conflict within myself about my response to motherhood is simple. As someone who has engaged with feminism mostly through my own life experiences, I have not experienced feminism through an academic lens. What I looked towards were the role models around me, women who I saw as empowered—strong, vocal, and successful women, who seemed to have it all together and who continued to grow professionally and contribute to the society, despite having children and a family to take care of. Before my own child started asserting himself in my womb, I had admired these women for their ability to dedicate themselves so completely to the cause (whatever the cause may be), despite the burden of managing their families. The women I had related to earlier had all modelled a different response to motherhood than the one I felt myself pulled towards. To my chagrin, I suddenly found myself questioning my earlier beliefs about what strong, feminist mothers should act like.

The strong, feminist mother modelled to me was one who still aced her career and made the right decisions for her child. She chose the right daycare, or the right nanny, and took pride in going back to work before the sanctioned maternity leave was over. This strong, feminist mom had me time; she had reading time and networking time. She was her own person. Her children were important, but they were more a part of her larger ecosystem than an essential part of herself. The feminist moms I saw around me hated the gender stereotyping and declared that they hated blue and pink. They lamented over the endless social messaging around girl roles and boy roles and shared tips about modelling nonstereotypical behaviour to the children.

But what most of these feminist moms didn't do was to accept choices other than the ones they were making as feminist ones. They scorned women who seemed to grow into new people with the arrival of their babies and pitied those whose identities became completely interlinked with their children

Across the majority of the feminist groups that I had been active in, the contempt towards women who chose to make motherhood their prime identity was obvious. Someone removed their own profile picture on Facebook and replaced it with one of their child? What is wrong with her? Whatever happened to her sense of self? What kind of a woman is she if her identity is primarily formed by a relationship? Before I was confronted with the emotional enormity of pregnancy and motherhood, this contempt had made perfect sense. Women were someone on their own after all and motherhood, no matter how cherished it is, is just a relationship in the end. It may be the most valuable relationship some women have, yet how sad that it is so all consuming that women seem to lose their sense of self.

But here I was in a state where my pregnancy and my child were slowly dominating each and every thought I had. Even though I pretended otherwise, I knew I had become one of those women—the ones I had previously seen with contempt and the ones who suddenly seemed to keep their work, careers, ambitions, and dreams at the fringes and centre their existence on the needs of their child. So every time I was reminded that a real conflict between family and work obligations had already begun, I became defensive. "It isn't that pregnant women can't travel of course," I'd write—refusing yet another invitation to a conference abroad, which would have been a high priority earlier—"It is just that my doctor doesn't feel very comfortable with the idea at this stage, given my age and my medical history. I can fly if it is very important, but without the doctor's certificate giving me the go ahead, the airlines won't book me on the flight. Such a shame!"

"I will take maternity leave of course," I'd tell my team when they asked me who would be my maternity cover. "But I'm always available on email. You know what kind of a workaholic I am. I'd die of boredom if I actually didn't work for three months." Every time I made one of those statements, I felt an unfamiliar sense of guilt rising within me and worked hard to ignore it. As a woman born in a South Asian, Muslim family, guilt is an automated response to anything that hints at conflict. My inability to give a hundred per cent to work as I previously had and my failure to commit a hundred per cent of my time to my growing family wrecked me emotionally. All of a sudden, it had become challenging for my professional and personal identities to coexist as they had done for years.

Whether I was ready or not, my identity was undergoing a primary shift. At the back of my mind, I knew I had to face the reality of this shift soon, but by the day the baby finally made his appearance, I had not really processed my thoughts.

*

We had simply gone in for a checkup that day; the due date was still a week away. I knew before the ultrasound was done that the baby was far from engaged—he had been kicking my ribs endlessly after all. There was some talk of induction if things remained the same next week, some routine talk, movement, energy levels, blah, blah, blah. But just as we got up to leave, my doctor asked me to get an ultrasound done before leaving the clinic, just to check the fluid level. I knew something was up the second the radiologist said, "Hmm, let me get your doctor." The fluid level was low, the cord was around his neck, and he was a bigger baby than we had previously thought. Back in the doctor's room, we listened as she said they'd have to induce urgently and explained the process of induction. She talked at length about why labour pains were more intense than those experienced during natural labour. I had done a ton of reading, but at that moment, I realized that my research had been too focused on how each process would affect the baby. I had no clear idea about how it would all affect me.

They all say that one has nine months to prepare oneself mentally for the arrival of a new baby. From the endless Mommy blogs I followed, simply to be with my child. I no longer get defensive and justify my lack of interest in working endless odd hours. I own the fact that I am not who I was, and being a different person now doesn't seem to be a betrayal to who I was.

I no longer see the changes in my own identity as nonfeminist choices. I am okay with how my identity is evolving. I say evolving because I know now that this process of growth as a parent is going to continue. Years down the road, I know that I will still be growing into motherhood.

Staying true to the feminist mold, I often find myself agonizing over the choices I make for my child. Some choices are easy. Nobody gets to tell him that boys don't cry (not even his grandparents who do believe that they shouldn't), and nobody gets to tell him that he should act like a man. He plays with cars and kitchen sets alike and gets more books than toys; he wears blue only as much as any other colour and wears pink with swag. He goes to the office with us and sees both Mama and Baba putting in the same hours at work and coming back to take care of home as a team.

These are the easy choices—choices one can make and feel self-congratulatory. And then there are choices that I know I should not be making—the decision to have him circumcised for instance. I could say that it wasn't a real choice for me after all. I live in a Muslim country, rife with violent conflict. I live in a country where religious intolerance grows by the day. And since I live here and belong to a Muslim family, saying no to something like circumcision, which is an essential part of a baby's initiation to the religion, would have put him at risk—the risk of social exclusion and bullying at best and actual violence at worst. The ideal choice would have been to wait till he was old enough to understand and give consent to having it done. Yet what would have happened in all the years in between? He might have been bullied, excluded, or isolated. How traumatic would it have been for him to get the procedure done as an adult?

There might be tougher choices to make still, as my growth into motherhood isn't just psychological. As I write this, I am pregnant with a little girl. This little girl will be born in a country where girls are still killed for honour and legislating against child marriages brings out protesting mobs to the streets. She will be born in a country where the majority believes that women are *naqis ul aqal*—creatures with flawed wisdom and should not be taken seriously. She will be born in a place where news of a six-year-old's rape and brutal murder is met by endless text messages containing religious advice about covering up little girls properly to ensure they don't tempt the pedophiles and remain safe.

What choices would I make to ensure that my little girl is safe in this place? And would these choices be the same choices that actually empower her? And would my choices for my son and my daughter be the same?

I don't really know yet.

To call oneself a proud feminist in a country like Pakistan is an immediate invitation for abuse. You are shunned for your supposedly Western ideals and seen as someone who is immoral. Your religious affiliation is questioned, and you are painted as either crazy or frustrated. As I grow into motherhood, my feminism makes me both strong and vulnerable at the same time. Can a feminist parent ever create a perfect balance between what is right in principle and what is safe on ground?

I do not know yet.

Chapter 13

Thinking and Practicing Parenting; or How to Do Right by My Child ... and Me

Elena Damma

Becoming a Parent: Reflections about Self and Others

When my daughter turned one year old, an acquaintance asked me if I shaved her hair because I did not want her to look like a girl. Perplexed, I asked her why she would think that. In all seriousness, she answered, "You remember how you told us not to buy you presents for your baby shower that would make her look like a girl, so I figured..." It was not difficult to remember that my colleague was referring to the fact that I had asked them not to buy her princess dresses. My wish to have my daughter wear a diverse range of clothes, not only stereotypical pink ones, was translated to me not wanting her to "look like a girl". It was, hence, logical to assume that I had shaved her hair for the same reason.

How to deal with societal expectations regarding visual representations of gender is only one of the many choices parents have to make on behalf of their children. Others include the way we encourage and support our children, the activities we encourage them to take up, how we discipline them, the expectations we place on them, and the way we make them understand these expectations. Others still concern the way we teach them about their identity, including their physical and behavioural boundaries, and how we teach them to define these for themselves.

Part of feminist parenting is the theorizing and the thinking, whereas the other part is the practical doing. In that vein, beyond attempting our best to educate our children, I believe that they learn from the way we live our lives as parents. When we have children, we do not suddenly acquire new identities as parents that are isolated from our identities as people. And I believe that the way we parent our children, beyond our conscious choices, is deeply rooted in who we are. Fundamentally, I believe that our parenting is informed by how we relate to other people, particularly to the ones who surround our children the most, including our children's other parents. As a white, European mother of a child whose father is a "local" in the African country we live in, and who arguably was socially and economically less well-positioned than me, I was privileged. This privilege was informed by many features, including gender, "race", culture, and class. Having lived with my daughter's father for many years before she was born, we were acutely aware of many of the implications that this intersectionality had on our lives. Although personal characteristics arguably shape some of the differences between individuals, I believe that our views on the most important aspects related to becoming parents and to parenting are largely influenced by socialization, education, and exposure, which act as a prism through which these intersections are reflected. Many parenting issues concern the question of who does what and why, and, hence, relate to ascribed rights, responsibilities, and duties in the family. Perceptions about who is in charge are deeply rooted in societal norms—particularly gender roles. I believe that one of the most complex aspects of social norms is that they inform our perception of normality. Whereas we are usually aware of our values or opinions, and able to define and defend them, we are often only partially conscious of our expectations of what is obvious and supposedly normal to us. Subjective normality is, thus, so difficult to negotiate because it typically manifests itself in the ways we act when our actions are not formed by conscious effort and when our "normal" clashes with someone else's "normal." Assumptions about normality in terms of responsibilities and decision making in parenting, for instance, manifest in how to ensure a healthy pregnancy, about the kind, place, and process of giving birth, about everyday care for the baby, about individual parent's activities and engagements outside of the family, about personal freedoms, and, crucially, about the redefinition of the couple. These assumptions also manifest in the big choices we make on behalf of our children, including matters related to religion, culture, and overall identity. Although both the big picture and the small picture decisions are fundamental for a family, parents often fail to negotiate their expectations and make conscious decisions about them because they assume that it is obvious how to go about them—until they clash. And most parents eventually do.

Defining Boundaries: Overcoming Social Norms and Imaginations of Self and Family

Despite having gone through many rough patches as a couple, my daughter's father and I had gotten used to overcoming our crises throughout the years. By the time I was due in October 2015, I thought we were prepared for our child. Conventional wisdom has it that the arrival of a child brings gender roles to the fore, which, in our case, translated to preconceived ideas and expectations about what it means to be a mother and a father, and ultimately about the rights, responsibilities, and duties of each of us. Often, the supposed innate ability of women to take care of their children is taken for granted—women give birth and, thus, most women are able to nurture their children. Considering the dependency of their child, most women have no choice but to ease into the role—some comfortably, others with a lot of difficulty—of becoming a mother. Many men, in contrast, whose immediate importance to their babies is perhaps not as tangible, seem to struggle to become parents. Although I reminded myself to be patient and to give my daughter's father time to somewhat grow into his new role, ostensibly without him ever wondering how I grew into mine, I witnessed him develop in a way that differed—literally violently—from my expectations.

My daughter's father and I have always had a complicated relationship. In hindsight, I often wonder why I did not end things with him before I finally did. There were too many red flags in our lives, broken promises, and broken dreams. Yet I hadn't taken the time, or mastered the strength, to really change my situation. We had built so much together and gone through so much together. The truth is also that I was so busy pursuing my professional life and attempting to have some balance with friends, women having to carry the entire mental load and sacrifice themselves for the sake of family unity. But I frankly had no idea how to deal with the situation. And I was so overwhelmed with resuming my fulltime job while expressing milk at the office three times a day and having the sole responsibility of caring for our daughter once I stepped into our home and relieved the nanny of their duties. I felt as if I did not even have space to breathe, let alone think or act.

One night, the opportunity to change my and my child's lives presented itself, and I grabbed it with both hands. That night, I returned from prolonged travel to attend a course at a Canadian university for three weeks. Since my daughter was barely seven months old at the time and I was still exclusively breastfeeding, I had secured a scholarship to travel with her and my mother as her caregiver. While taking a course that brought together a wide range of activists and professionals with a passion for dignified, agency-based development from all over the world, I experienced a feeling of community that overwhelmed and inspired me. I was both touched and shocked by how people whom I had never met before could be so much more present, interested, and supportive than the man who called himself my family. After our graduation, I got sick and had to postpone my flight home for a few days. Pressured to return to my work as soon as possible, and barely healthy enough to travel, I finally took a flight home, alone with my daughter. That night, I had to wait for him to pick us up at the airport for an hour with my sleeping daughter strapped to my belly, barely strong enough to stand. When we finally got home, there was no food at all. Our house was dusty and had not been cleaned in a long time. And the bedsheets were still the same ones I had left six weeks earlier, including hers, which were even soiled. He responded with cheap excuses to my shock and terror. That night, I knew that nothing in the world could excuse or justify how little he cared for us—and my not stepping up for myself and my daughter.

Shaken by his most recent display of indifference and completely uncertain about how to deal with the situation, I proposed to move out of our home with our daughter; I was still hopeful that the physical distance would help us to become more mindful about each other and our new roles as parents. Her father, in the meantime, seemed neither keen on seeing her nor interested in taking any kind of responsibility for her, or for me. He hardly came to see us, and when he did come, he often came close to her bedtime and was often drunk. On several occasions, he became rowdy and threatened both me and the child, and I had to call on neighbours to get him out of my apartment. Our situation deteriorated quickly. It went from trying to free myself from a destructive relationship, while attempting to maintain a space for my daughter to be with her father, to having to question what I needed to do to make sure she was emotionally and physically safe. I was compelled to share intimate and painful details of my life with the security manager at my work place and even the police. And yet, I continued to be uncertain about what to do.

Due to my own upbringing, having both a mother and father around when growing up was normal for me and, hence, desirable. I did not want my own hurt feelings and disappointments to interfere with my daughter's choices. At the same time, I also had to acknowledge that it was up to me to protect her from getting hurt. But what does that really mean? It was an especially relevant question, since her father continued to deny the negative impact he had on both of us and continued paying lip service to loving his child. What more did I need? He loved his child. He loved his child, right? They say actions speak louder than words, and his actions did not entail a trace of love for her but a trail of neglect. After a particularly violent night, it started dawning on me that I could no longer remain stuck in inaction and hide behind not wanting to keep her father away from her; I had no choice but to make decisions on her behalf. I had to protect her and myself. And I had to let go of the idea of his being part of her life.

Affirming Feminist Principles in Life and in Parenting as a Single Mother

Scared but elated by my newly found strength, I started facing life as a single, foreign mother in my daughter's father's country of origin, far away from my own family who could have provided us with structure and a place where we belonged. So I had no choice but to make it a home for both of us. Our situation had various practical, ethical, and also legal implications. And I had to confront all of them. Some of the practical implications involved deciding who would care for her, which school she would go to, or whom she would socialize with. It also involved finding ways to raise my child to explore, know, and embrace her mixed roots and, hence, deciding which cultures, religions, and languages I taught her as being hers. One of the things of primary concern to me, in that context, was how to teach her about her Africanness without engaging in cultural appropriation and without distancing her from her localness by taking up too much space in defining her identity, which would push her in the role of a bystander, excluded by my foreignness and my relative privilege.

Being a foreigner in our country of residence also had legal implications, which forced me to seek painstaking legal redress. The most appalling part was that despite being her mother, I had no right to remove my daughter from the country's territory without her father's consent. At the same time, having a child who bears the nationality of my host country, alongside my own, does not grant me residence, or even a visa. Since my country of residence has a reputation for corrupt civil servants attempting to benefit from personal miseries, and due to the fact that white women figure among top-suspects for child trafficking in this region, I was very worried about involving the authorities. My embassy's warning that it would be child abduction if I left the country with her made me understand that there was no other way out. I had tried to settle things with him out of court through my lawyer. But he refused any kind of consensus, any kind of agreement. After months of weighing options, I decided to take him to court. Against my expectations, the judge granted me custody of my child alongside freedom of movement.

Despite everything I had gone through, I continued to find myself exposed to prejudice and accusations of having failed in my presumed womanly responsibilities to maintain my household at any cost, including by some of the people whom I had counted as close friends. One of these supposed friends even called my mother and told her to make me drop the court case, or else he would have me killed, adding "you know, this is Africa." Beyond everything else, the loneliness in my empty apartment, far away from the neighbourhood in which we used to live, was crushing me after having shared our house with friends and family for years.

Being a single parent is difficult. And having so much power over my daughter's life is terrifying at times. How to deal with her father, who will always continue to be part of her, has been one of the toughest decisions I have continuously had to make—about her level of involvement with him, how to portray him, and how to verbalize his absence. After cutting him out completely for almost a year, I have allowed him to see her several times in the past months, and it was ok. Above all, she seemed happy.

How to engage other significant persons—including the man whom I slowly understand as my new partner—in her life is another important matter. Some persons in our environment offer mostly unsolicited advice and caution me to ensure that she knows the difference between her father and my new partner, who has been caring for her much more than her biological father. Obviously, many people assume that being a father is a position acquired solely through transmission of genes, hence excluding those whose fatherhood is defined by love and dedication rather than biology. Others push me to "reestablish harmony" so as to "allow her to grow up in an intact family"—somewhat encouraging me to subjugate my decisions and my sense of temporality to my presumed responsibility to provide her with an ideal-typical family structure, even if it does not involve her biological father. Although I deeply wish that my daughter grows up in a house of love, togetherness, and family, I remain aware that some of the most important things I want to teach my child are freedom of choice, a right to happiness, and the understanding that life does not always go as planned. Specifically, I want to teach her that being a woman does not automatically imply having to do more, accept more, but get less. I want her to know that her wishes, interests, and preferences are legitimate, no matter what. I hence try to resist my socially acquired and deeply internalised urge to reestablish balance and try to allow my personal disequilibrium to inspire me to choose a path for myself at my own pace; I do not allow other people to define the "right" way of going about my situation or to subdue my personal life to the presumed needs of my child. I know I may make a lot of mistakes along the way, but I try to do me and her justice, and I hope that one day, she will understand. Ultimately, I remain convinced that my strength will make her stronger and that my having an identity outside of motherhood empowers me to better take care of, as well as protect, my daughter. And I continue to believe that the most important role we play as parents is to live our lives in a way that we hope our children will live theirs one day—unapologetic, authentic, and passionate. Although this is certainly true for any parent, it matters to me that she learns that a woman can do whatever she sets her mind to do and that she should not allow anything to prevent her from living in her truth.

Thinking and Practicing Feminist Parenting: A Few Lessons Learned

Reflecting about my experience, I think that I learned invaluable lessons about both parenting as a process and about how we can support other parents. Being a parent is difficult, and we will make many mistakes throughout our children's lives; some of them will be genuine because we do not know better, but most of them will be because we are tired, overwhelmed, and impatient—because we are human. And that's ok. Whenever I feel that I have failed my daughter, I remind myself to be patient and forgiving with myself. She has to learn that people are not always perfect, that people make mistakes, and that they can get angry, but that they still love her. I also believe that it is important to accept the responsibility of being ourselves and of learning how to negotiate ourselves, flaws and all, with our children. In the same vein, I also consciously resist the urge to cover up how I feel. Although I am careful not to expose her to the depth of those feelings, I believe that it is important for her to learn that people cannot always be happy but that they get better as well.

Asking for and accepting help, as a single mom particularly, are other important things that I have had to learn. I cannot always do everything on my own. And that's ok, too. Having a loving caregiver with whom my daughter spends most of her time on weekdays has been invaluable for me. Luckily, it is the absolute norm in my host country that families across the social spectrum have house help and that most children are coraised by nannies from a tender age. Although having someone in charge of my daughter whom I have to employ obviously implies that our relationship is hierarchical, despite our good connection, and entails a plethora of complexities, I also work on resisting the urge to micromanage people who take charge of her. Despite there being some important ground rules, I believe that children feel whether someone is their authentic self or not. And I want my daughter to learn how to interact and deal with different people, as well as their character and their ways of doing things. By letting my nanny be herself—and by encouraging her to treat my daughter "normally" and to raise her according to her own standards—having a local caregiver also provides me with a crucial opportunity to give my daughter access to her own localness. This is ultimately also why I have continued to pursue the possibility for her to safely meet and interact with her father. I also encourage her to explore him in herself as much as possible rather than attempting to shield her and forbid her from wanting to see her father's reflection in herself. At the same time, I continue trying to protect her from his difficult sides while remaining vigilant not to transfer my pain and my disappointments to her and not to ever make her feel as if she must choose between him and me. Despite everything, he is her father, and I want to allow her to love, cherish, and admire him if she wishes to, but I also plan to be as honest and fair in my conversation with her about what happened when she is old enough to ask about it.

With other children's questions about her father's whereabouts, seeing fathers in books, and meeting her friends' fathers, my daughter clearly understands the normative belief that a father should be part of a family. The power of labelling things and people struck me the day that I decided to tell her that the man whom she had just met for the first time in months was her daddy. Seeing her face light up, exclaiming "I want daddy," I felt at peace with my decision. Despite hardly seeing him, I observe that knowing that she has a daddy, just like her friends, gives her peace. At the same time, I also try to be confident that children grow up more healthily when they are raised and surrounded by people who are healthy and happy. So, I am consciously allowing myself to pursue my personal happiness and to date without holding myself to societal standards of how and what family is supposed to be. While accepting to make a space for her biological father in her life, I try to show her that surrounding yourself with loving other significant persons is great, too. Building, accepting, and sustaining solidarities with different people independently of their label is an important part of an emotionally, psychologically, and socially healthy life. In the same vein, I also do not restrict her too much in terms of whom she socializes with. It requires a lot of small and sometimes painful acts of letting go and relinquishing control, especially when I feel that others exoticize her, for instance by wanting to touch her hair and skin. At the same time, I want her to develop a sense of what she is comfortable with and how to deal with people in her space from an early age.

Another completely different but important issue in the context of supporting her self-determination concerns how I teach her about food and eating. Having grown up in Europe, where most women have complicated relationships with food and body image issues, I am trying to foster a healthy relationship between her, her body, and food. I see

Chapter 14

It Takes a Village, as Long as You Have One

OluTimehin Adegbeye

Throughout my childhood and before I became a mother, my extended family was, besides being mostly newly and nominally religious, what most people would describe as close. There were three living generations descended from or related to my grandfather who spent a lot of time together at my grandparents' house, and celebrations like New Year's Day, weddings, and birthdays filled the rooms and gardens with people and laughter.

For the most part, the units formed in my mother's generation by marriage and birth were distinct from the whole, but only to the degree to which we defined one another as cousins or uncles and aunts. The only relatives we didn't feel a close bond with lived either in Northern Nigeria or in England, and even then, we visited them as often as we could. For those family members who lived in our base of Lagos, Nigeria, the work of raising my generation was distributed on the basis of opportunity and expertise among the adults. As such, for most of my life, "family" was a collective concept—a large group of people whose shared blood fostered goodwill and support.

My grandmother, who had a background in education, conducted or supervised after-school lessons for any of the grandchildren who needed them. Discipline and correction could be meted out by any adult, but the most egregious cases were reserved for my mother and grandfather. (I wager this was because of their impressive ability to unperturbedly watch recalcitrant adolescents beg for mercy, as they stood with trembling muscles on one leg with their arms spread.) Affection was freely given and freely received by the children, and on Sundays after church, my grandfather would pile us into one of his Mercedes Benz cars to go buy ice cream. To my childhood self, it was a happy and mostly safe family, and its conservatism was not apparent to me because I existed within its confines.

Growing up, the implications of gender were rarely readily apparent to me. I was quick-witted and humorous in a way that the adults—especially my grandfather and mother—encouraged. I was a star student, an athlete, and an active churchgoer, eventually becoming a teen leader. My biggest failing was my utter dislike of cooking—a feeling that not even the much-bemoaned hunger pangs of my future husband and children could change. Then I got pregnant out of wedlock in my final year of university and chose not to terminate the pregnancy, and for the first time in my life, I was firmly outside of the boundaries of what my family considered acceptable female conduct.

My grandfather had passed away ten years before my pregnancy, and my mother had been holding the family together by managing his estate and doing the emotional labour of maintaining the kinship bond. Because I had never noticed the patriarchal lines along which my family organized itself, it did not occur to me that her leadership and power within the family might be considered unusual. Despite her being the second child and female, her being in charge was simply what was sensible. She was in a similar line of work to grandpa—the one with whom he enjoyed the closest relationship following the death of his favourite of his two sons—and she alone had functioning relationships with all of her siblings outside of the collective camaraderie. In retrospect, I realize that this was not because my family didn't quite 'do gender', but because my *mother* didn't.

In our nuclear family, my mother was also the anchor. My father was abusive and mentally ill—albeit not necessarily in that order. My relationships to my siblings and father mostly radiated out from my and their relationship to my mother; she was a stabilizing force, our centre of gravity. After I had my daughter, people often asked why I didn't get an abortion since the procedure is quite common in Nigeria despite being illegal. I would respond by saying "because I knew my family would support me no matter what." Like with the gender question, I didn't realize until much later that what I meant was "I knew my mother would support me no matter what." To a certain extent my mother, while she was alive, embraced feminist politics out of necessity. The circumstances of her marriage and career made it such that she simply could not afford to settle into conservative womanly roles, even if she had been so inclined—which she wasn't.

My mother, who was secretly ill with cancer, died when I was six months pregnant. Until the day it happened, it never occurred to me that she could die, even though in the two weeks we spent together prior to her death, I saw her sicker and weaker than I ever had before. I was in school finishing the first semester of my final year, and my sister later informed me that mummy didn't tell me much because she felt that my pregnancy was upheaval enough. While I was away at school I had no idea how ill she was or even that she had cancer. She called me every other day, texted me on her Blackberry more than she ever had before, and showered me with love. I thought it was because I was pregnant and scared. In conversations with my sister after her passing, it became clear that it was also because she was dying and afraid for me.

Contrary to what most people around me believe due to the trope of the "single mother who overcomes great odds," the great difficulty of my life was not becoming an unwed mother—it was losing my own mother in the same breath. Suddenly, I was in the world without the maternal protection I had taken for granted, and it was not long before the cracks started to show. I hadn't realized that my mother had been almost alone in bearing the responsibility of keeping our family a community or that people within the collective had taken our cues on how to treat one another from her. She had been the central figure with whom they had a long history of love and trust; she was the only one able or willing to do the work of tempering excesses or dampening the hunger to gain and wield power over my grandfather's wealth and other family members. She was the only one whose life was an undeniable example of female power, autonomy, and leadership.

I don't doubt that my mother's fear for my future was connected to her knowledge of what lay behind the shield she had been for me. My mother inherited her father's no-nonsense, pragmatic, and clear-minded decisiveness; it allowed her to recognize the existence of obstacles just so that she could surmount them. Because she routinely flew in the face of gendered illogic by simply existing and excelling at the intersection of opportunity and expertise, she was the type of woman people called a man as a compliment. Furthermore, any backlash her unyielding nature might have generated was tempered by her clear devotion to her husband and marriage: she was a virtuous woman, dedicated to her God and her man. Her willfulness was, thus, forgivable. Unfortunately, in passing down family traits, my mother endowed me with her iron will but somehow neglected to pass down the faith or fidelity that made her stubbornness easier to swallow. As such, her willfulness was forgivable; mine has never been.

In the historical Oyo Yorùbá world-sense, as described by Oyèwùmí, Oyèrónké in her seminal work *What Gender Is Motherhood?*, there is no higher status than that of Iya—the mother. Conceived as both a biological and spiritual role, motherhood and mothering conferred an unquestionable, fixed seniority—and, thus, immense social value—on the mother. The birth of children was constructed as divine in the society; children were received as the ultimate objective of life itself, and the raising of children was considered a collective effort of utmost importance. Questions of marital status and the paternity of children were secondary considerations, which could not impinge upon motherhood status and which did not significantly affect the support offered to the mother or the care received by the child.

However, this mindset barely survived the incursion of colonization or its deliberate delegitimization of local ways of thinking, which favoured hierarchical and dehumanizing logics. The combination of patriarchal subjugation of people understood to be women, a perverted insistence on regulating consensual sexual contact, and the promotion of monogamous, church- and state-sanctioned heterosexual marriage as the only valid outlet for (men's) sexual desire proved lethal. Almost inexorably, the concept of the legitimacy of children—and by extension, of motherhood—took hold.

Because the birth of children outside of wedlock results in immediate devaluation of young women (making abuse of said young women even more acceptable than the norm), young unwed mothers in Nigeria often leave the responsibility of raising their children to their own mothers, with the children frequently believing their birth mothers to be their siblings. Pregnant young women are also often hastily married to the father in order to restore some sort of respectability to the mother, child and family.

My daughter was born amid my family's unchecked collapse into flagrant patriarchal conservatism. Or perhaps the birth of a female child to me, an unmarried young woman, in the absence of my mother simply provided an avenue for what had always been there to reveal itself. In any case, we were the easiest and most logical targets for filial recalibration. First, my grandmother's siblings tried to manipulate the father of my child into marrying me at a family meeting, to which my body but not my input was invited. After perhaps an hour of being carefully chided for his role in devaluing me as a potential wife to someone else, my daughter's father mentioned that he had repeatedly asked me to marry him and I said no. My great-uncles and aunts looked at me properly for the first time, their faces contorted in confused shock. The meeting dissolved into chaos when I confirmed the claim, and I was shepherded outside so they could convince themselves that I didn't know what I was saying.

My refusal to marry the man was not a feminist decision, not in any conscious way at least. But I had known even while sleeping with him that I didn't want a future with him; getting pregnant due to a convergence of inadequate sex education and failed coitus interruptus had not changed that. I had taken for granted that my family would be there for me in the same way it always had, so I was oblivious to the whisperings and grumblings that surrounded my pregnancy. I was completely ignorant of the great upset that was my having brought my grandmother's first great-grandchild into the world without having first been transferred into the ownership of a man via marriage, but my obliviousness was only natural. My grandmother had jumped to her feet and danced when I told her the news. My mother had asked me, somewhat rhetorically and with a voice full of sadness, "how did it happen?" and then she had taken me to buy amala when that was all I wanted to eat. To me and the women who raised me, my pregnancy was merely a bump in the road, so it did not occur to me that other people saw it as a full stop and resented me for not feeling the same.

Over the years, I slowly learned how naive I was, how unwed mothering in my society is in many ways an exercise in navigating abuse, and how much of that abuse comes from within the family. My mother was a single mother for several years after she kicked my father out for his violence, but she did such an excellent job of shielding us from the social impacts of that decision that it never occurred to me that there was something wrong with single motherhood. Thus, the expectation that young women who have children out of wedlock must perform shame and offer their lives up to be controlled by external parties, especially their families, was new and quite absurd to me. I also resented the fact that because I had gotten pregnant by accident, I was perceived to be totally and permanently irresponsible and, worse, incapable of directing my own life or making important decisions about my child and her care.

My awakening to feminist politics coincided neatly with my daughter's infancy, and in the first year of her life, I decided that I wanted to raise my child as free of abuse as possible. To me, this meant not hitting her, not talking down at her, not trying to control her, not shaming her about her body, and not promoting harmful gendered ideas in her upbringing. I wanted her to feel even freer to explore the world and claim space in it than my mother had made it possible for me to feel. I observed how differently people treated her when they thought she was a boy (which, until fairly recently, happened often). Noticing how much more open people were to her high energy and mischief when they misgendered her made it even more important to me to find ways to circumvent their predispositions towards limiting her due to her gender.

My feminist politics also informed a strong aversion to the way in which children's choices and bodies are violently policed in Nigeria, such that any evidence of autonomy or will is treated as disobedience or insolence deserving of severe punishment. Also of particular concern were the ways in which people minimized or dismissed inappropriate physical contact and sexual misconduct or abuse, despite or even because of how pervasive it is in this country. Finally, I was committed to maintaining my identity as an independent individual, alongside my motherhood status. My desire was to be a good mother and a fulfilled person, so I continued to pursue personal happiness to the best of my ability. Unfortunately, I didn't realize quite how costly these ideas and decisions would be. I didn't know that my clear-mindedness about what I wanted for myself and my child would be received as arrogance and disruptiveness deserving of violent pushback.

As a feminist, I am committed to rejecting patriarchal ideas in their entirety. My mothering is led and guided by my child's individual needs and development rather than by externally dictated norms. It is crucial to me that my child understands that "girl" can mean something different to her than it does to the rest of our society. This is why I encourage her freedom by modelling the same at whatever cost. This is why I indulge her curiosity, her pleasure, and her awareness of her body as a vehicle that must be cared for rather than a gilded cage from which she must regard an undiscoverable world. I refuse to teach my child to shrink herself. I also refuse to send her the message that her version of the world must be a shrunken one in order for her to be safe. I encourage her to trust her own mind and intuition by validating what she thinks and feels. I try to remain open to the lessons she offers me in how to live with kindness and integrity, and I teach her about her own power to shape the world by telling her stories about powerful women, including her grandmother.

If patriarchy is the logic of social organization, then anyone who rejects patriarchy is a threat to social order. By the time my daughter was two, the treatment I received at the hands of my family and other older adults who had been part of my life through my mother had deteriorated significantly, especially as it became increasingly clear that I was intent on choosing the course of my life regardless of social norms or pressure. The support I received upon my daughter's birth was slowly and systemically withdrawn in the wake of each of my so-called transgressions. I was punished, in various ways, for each deviation from the path of repentance or respectability: refusing to marry; failing to display that I was ashamed and had learned my lesson by abandoning a social life and my male friends in particular; entering into a new romantic and sexual relationship when my daughter was eight months old; refusing to end that relationship simply because my family considered it improper; getting birth control; abandoning Christianity, etc.

I was asked to move out of the home of the relatives who took me in after my mother's death and my daughter's birth because they felt that I might corrupt their teenage daughter. Family members made this decision despite being fully aware that my daughter was only five or six months old. I was earning a pittance at my first job—my daughter's father was not supporting us financially or otherwise—and the only housing option available to me at the time was my late mother's home, where my brother and mentally ill, treatment-averse father lived, who also had a well-known history of physical violence.

About a year after my aunt asked me to leave her home at her husband's behest, an older family friend who was considered an aunt physically assaulted me, locked me in her home for two days, and seized my mobile devices because I had left Christianity and also refused to end the romantic relationship that was one of my few sources of comfort and support at the time. When I made it clear that even if I ended the relationship, I would not be returning to church, she told me "sinners" were not welcome in her home.

I was forced to move back into my mother's house, despite knowing it was potentially unsafe for me and my child. Unfortunately, my mostly good relationship with my brother, who also lived there with his family, then began to deteriorate almost in direct (inverse) proportion to my levels of certainty about what I did and didn't want for my daughter and myself. He increasingly saw no problem with crossing my personal or parenting boundaries; he would shame and verbally abuse me for not cooking for or cleaning up after him, or attempt to convince me that I deserved to be unhappy for having a child out of wedlock. He also made serious threats of physical violence on more than one occasion, including in front of my toddler, for reasons such as my having gone on a weekend getaway with my then boyfriend (while my daughter was safe with my sister), my refusal to let him hit my child as discipline, or my refusal to let him intimidate a male visitor of mine.

My brother, despite having been raised almost exclusively by women in general and my mother in particular, ended up being one of the first-line enforcers of patriarchal control in my family. It was increasingly apparent as I became more serious about the boundaries of his influence in my or my child's life that there was no physical, emotional, or psychological harm that he was not willing to threaten or commit in order to demonstrate my subordinate status in the family and in society. I eventually severed all ties with him when in an argument that started because he refused to take instructions about my mother's company from my older sister since he "could never defer to a woman," he tried to silence me by screaming that I "hated men" because I had been raped.

After this incident, I moved away to my grandmother's already crowded house with my then two-year-old daughter. I thought it would be safe for both of us because it was the same house I had spent so much time in as a happy and mostly unencumbered child. Unfortunately, I was forced to move out again not long after when I found out that one of the distant relatives also living in the house had sexually abused multiple children. I was horrified to learn that several members of my family were aware of this and my aunt had, in fact, taken one of his victims to the hospital, but no one considered it necessary either to enforce consequences for his actions or to inform me so that I could limit his access to my child. When I confronted the aunt who had taken this teenaged abuser's victim to the hospital, she asked me to "give him the benefit of the doubt." All of these incidents reified the idea I already had: my family—like many families in conservative, hyper-religious Nigeria—is in many ways inherently unsafe for women and girls, and to parent my child safely and in safety, I would need to distance myself from them.

In navigating the minefield that my family became in the wake of motherhood, feminism has been a double-edged sword. Early on, it provided me with the tools to recognize the ways in which my abilities and experiences were delegitimized because I was an unwed mother. It helped me to envision and enact ways of loving my child that validate and protect her. But it also reinforced my new social location as an unruly and transgressive woman, which made the withdrawal of support and protection justifiable to those who should have offered it. Still, being able to parent my child in this way—rather than accepting harm for choosing to be a mother or allowing my child to be exposed to abuse—is worth it to me. I believe it is better to be without blood family than to capitulate to ideas of fictive kinship that require me to accept ongoing violence while indirectly teaching my child that this is what it means to be a woman in the world.

Parenting in this way has taken a toll that rarely offers relief besides the reward of watching my daughter thrive, especially since like much of my own family, her other blood parent generally chooses not to contribute meaningfully to the effort. Not only have I had to parent with the support of no family members except my sister, I have also had to dedicate a good amount of my emotional energy to protecting both my child and myself from my family's harm. Without my mother, whose presence would have acted as both shield and source of support, my family is no longer a safe place, and my need for support, community, and guidance has been treated as negotiable or secondary by the people who would ordinarily be my first port of call. If mothering is generosity and if mothering requires giving, nurturing, and depletion, where do young unmarried women who often come to motherhood scared and doubting themselves go for replenishment?

Unfortunately, as long as Nigerian families remain unquestioningly founded on Eurocentric ideas of marriage and hierarchical gender relations, as long as kinship is organized around notions of love that cannot exist without domination, and as long as women's status within the family is conditional upon our silence in the face of abuse and our willingness to conform to social norms that hurt us, it will be safer for mothers like me to parent outside of the family. Thus, I have evolved away from my childhood idea of family as a blood-based tie. Instead, my goal is now to envision and build a family community for myself and my child that does not require, in exchange for its support, my bruised and bloodied acquiescence to our dehumanization.

Instead of my blood family, I look to the communities of women that I have found and created for support, guidance, and healing comfort when things get difficult. In teaching my daughter that "girl" can mean whatever she wants it to, and in grieving and honouring my mother who made "woman" whatever she wanted it to be, I am fashioning "family" into what I need it to be: a place of safety and love—at any cost, no matter what.

Works Cited

Oyèwùmí, Oyèrónké, *What Gender Is Motherhood: Changing Yorùbá Ideals of Power, Procreation, and Identity in the Age of Modernity.* Palgrave MacMillan, 2016.

Chapter 15

Feminism, Mothering, and Choice

Angelica Sorel

The idea of mother as primary care-giver is embodied in ideals of motherhood in many societies, including mine. Feminism presents itself to us as about choice. But when it comes to motherhood, how much scope is there for women in heterosexual relationships to take up the ideals of autonomy, freedom, and choice, and elect not only to share care with another but to defer to their parenting as primary? If we think about primary caregiving as a reproductive choice in itself for women, rather than simply as consequent to making the choice to have children, what does this imply for a feminist approach to parenting?

In this chapter, I reflect on some of these questions. I explore the cultural assumptions that I internalized as a white European middle-class woman in a heterosexual relationship, as I contemplated having children. I narrate the shock of having my first child, what becoming a mother did to my identity and sense of self, and the ways in which this began to erode the equality of a heterosexual—and deliberately nonmarital—relationship that had been carefully built on ideals of mutuality and gender neutrality. I go on to reflect on what kind of mother that made me and to the process of conscientization through which I began to apply my feminist anthropological knowledge to my own life. I examine how this process changed my experience of my relationships, not only with my children but also with their father. In telling the story of these choices, I reflect on the intentionality of these actions and on questions of agency, representation, and consciousness.

Motherhood Choices

Before I became a mother, I had never considered the possibility that stepping into and out of a status, role, and identity as primary caregiver once I'd given birth was a choice. Nor did I conceive of it being one that I could choose to make. In the narratives on motherhood with which I grew up surrounded by narratives on motherhood in which there was little space for the kind of mother who had a life in which other things, other work, and other people might also be important, let alone one that involved preserving some degree of freedom. These visions of motherhood did not contain within them the possibility of genuinely shared responsibility, let alone ceding the role of primary caregiver to someone else. Choosing to have a child seemed to be an all-or-nothing transition from a life in which I could decide and do what I wanted to one in which the child or children would have primacy—forever.

Like so many women of my race, sexuality, class and generation, I'd been raised with images of heterosexual motherhood that were all about being there: being the one with whom the principal responsibilities for one's child(ren) lay, being at home when the children came back from school, and being the one who nurtured and administered the hugs and kisses to mend bruised limbs or feelings. I had no role models for any other way of being or doing motherhood. At work, I was part of a social group of feminist colleagues with spectacularly successful careers, who were also very much in command of the kitchen, children and home. Liberal maternalism infused my workplace, expressed in the form of concessions given to women who became mothers so they could attend to their children and complaints when such accommodations were rendered difficult to ask for or not given. I was surrounded by those who valorized women's part-time *work*, but not women's part-time *mothering*. I knew of no men who went part-time to look after their children, gave their excuses to leave meetings early to pick up their children, or avoided or cut short international travel because of their caring responsibilities. I took it all in, unthinkingly.

Feminism should have lent me a different perspective. I remember the revelation of reading Felicity Edholm, Olivia Harris, and Kate Young's 1979 piece, which made the powerful argument that there is nothing necessary about the work of social reproduction that attaches it to a female body, let alone to a mother; this work of caring can and is done by others. By separating into three parts the acts of giving birth and breastfeeding, the work of bringing up children, the labour of maintaining the family, and the reproduction of the social, they helped me see as a feminist possibility a genuinely shared approach to parenting. This dislocation of the biological and the social should have permitted me to see other possibilities, including that of becoming one of many carers without privileging my own role in that relationship of care.

The literature on feminist mothering draws on a distinction between motherhood as *status* and mothering as *practice*, inspired by Adrienne Rich (1976). Motherhood is problematized for the normative ideals that it encodes, whereas mothering is cast as a way in which feminists can enact practices that challenge those ideals and, with it, contest and transform patriarchal social norms and arrangements (Gordon; O'Reilly). Feminist mothering—which I interpret as carrying feminist ideals of equality, autonomy, and freedom into the practice of mothering—offers the possibility of redefining motherhood for ourselves and inhabiting it as a site of resistance (O'Reilly; Horwitz). But to do so is, almost by definition, counter-cultural. I have come to see becoming a feminist mother as an unfolding, contested and messy process rather than a neatly defined identity that can simply be selected and taken up. In the complex mix of personal and political, there are also the biographical, generational, cultural and situational dimensions of mothering as practice and motherhood as status.

I go on to explore these dilemmas through an autobiographical narrative from a positionality as a white, middle-class, mostly heterosexual British woman. I begin by reflecting on the disjuncture between what I thought I was getting into and what actually happened when I first became a mother. I go on to narrate the process through which I reclaimed my presence in the workplace and then began to think, again, about what equality and gender neutrality in parenting might actually look like. From there, I examine the assumptions that I gradually brought into closer examination and sought to shake off, and how that transformed my relationship with my own mothering identity and practice. In this piece, my focus is not on my children but on my own experience of becoming and being what I considered to be a *feminist parent*. I conclude by reflecting back what my children, now teenagers, tell me about their experience of having me as a mum and what this taught them about gender, power, and love.

both our surnames. It was an elegant solution—one that at the same time evoked a political writer whose words captured the essence of what had brought us together. How much more romantic could you get than that?

But romance was not part of this particular decision, at least for him, and especially for his parents. It was all about lineage—his family name, his seed, his legacy. I refused to register the birth until we'd come to consensus. Three weeks later, we trooped down to the registry office and with an ink fountain pen, I signed the compromise. He got his last name. I got my last name as the last-but-one name, reasoning that a bit of give and take might just buy me the peace to not have a terrible thing to hold against me forever. And, as part of the compromise, I slipped into the middle the beautiful name I'd wanted my son, and later my daughter, to have.

That act of compromise marked a turning point of sorts. I became conscious that this was, and would be, a battle. My ostensibly liberal-minded partner was, however unconsciously, reproducing the very values that as a feminist I was preoccupied with changing. And that's where the rebellion was seeded. It didn't feel like that for the long, dark weeks of mothering that unfolded from the moment that I was able to walk again and watch him resume a busy and exciting working life. He'd come home and I'd say, tell me about your day, and he'd say, "Oh it was just meetings." Meetings, I'd think, how interesting to be meeting with people, talking ideas, and doing something of substance. My days went by in a blur of dealing with a screaming and sleepless child and deadly boring conversations with other mothers about sleep, nappies and poo. *Tell me about your interesting meetings*, I'd think, *and I'll try not to tell you about how miserable my day was*. The awfulness of the days didn't lift. I'd taught myself to be like Pollyanna and find one thing to be happy about, no matter what. I couldn't find a single positive thing, a single happy moment in many of my days. They were gruelling, tedious, lonely. I cried a lot. I shopped to ease the sadness. My partner would complain about how much money I was spending. *His* money. I was reduced to utter dependency.

It was only later that I admitted to myself that I'd lied when they gave me a questionnaire to fill in to assess whether I was suffering from postnatal depression, thinking that if I showed just how miserable I really was, I would have failed the test. The thought strayed into my mind in my darker moments that I might end up on medication or, worse, having my baby taken away. I was so sleep deprived that I had lost any sense of myself, my agency, and my rights. Everyone said "enjoy your baby." I wasn't enjoying my baby. I wasn't enjoying anything. I wanted to be having those meetings. I knew I wouldn't find them boring. I wanted to be having conversations about how to change the world rather than blotting out the tedium with chat about breastfeeding and nappies. And all my baby did was scream. He howled in the evening. He yelled in the night. He'd have a temporary lull, and I'd fall, exhausted, into a deep sleep, then be wrenched out of it and it would begin again. He couldn't bear me to put him down, so I didn't. Days could pass without me even managing to get dressed and out of the house.

Working Mother

When I was pregnant, I'd gone for a job interview. With my ripe belly bursting through the trousers of my suit, I never thought they'd give me the position. What more of a liability than a woman pregnant with her first child? But they did. My boss was impatient for me to begin. I said, "Look, I need a bit of time. I don't know how I'll feel once the baby is born." He said, "Look, we have a big grant and a huge opportunity. I want you on the team." I ended up going back to work when my baby was four months old, part time. I'd take him to workshops and pass him around while I presented or facilitated. Once, perilously close to the time when I was due to talk on a plenary panel at a large conference, he filled the air with an unmistakeable odour. I whisked him off to the toilet, changed his nappy, thrust him in the lap of my boss, and strode onto the stage. My boss commented later on how stunned he was at the seamless segue. It was not as effortless as it looked.

Female colleagues had lent me the wisdom that hiring a nanny was the least stressful way out of the juggling act. It seemed a good idea to spend my wages on someone to be with my son rather than face the stress of rushing to pick him up from the nursery or having to have days off work when he had a cold or diarrhoea, which, other mothers told me, happens all the time when babies go to nurseries. I'm not sure why I thought it was my responsibility to do all this, but it was somehow impressed upon me that mothering involved me being the one to drop or miss work. It seems hard to imagine now, too, where I got the idea that being seen to be professional required that I went home three times during each working day to breastfeed. My son never did take a bottle. We tried. We failed. Even the nanny failed, and she was a professional. I'd drive at breakneck speed, my breasts spilling over with milk, arrive to his screams, feed and change him, and then race back to work.

My office was my sanctuary. It was the first time I'd ever had an office of my own. It had my name on the door. And when the door was closed with me and only me inside the office, I experienced a feeling of joy. It was my space. At first, I was on a 50 per cent contract, something that I can't recall ever actively desiring—a default decision chosen in response to moral pressure not to work fulltime. After about a year, I increased my hours to 75 per cent. I wasn't quite sure how much was expected of me at 75 per cent, but it felt like a good enough compromise; it was almost fulltime, but still part-time enough to make a nod to the expectation that as a mother I should not actually want to be at work fulltime. It felt as if there was something unnatural, almost indecent, about spending my time at the office out of choice rather than spending every minute tending to my child. But work had lifted me out of my depressive gloom, opening up to me new vistas. It was exhilarating, if rather overwhelming—especially on less than two hours uninterrupted sleep a night. I craved it like a drug.

A female colleague, the only senior female figure in the organization, took me aside. She knew how the place worked and that women who were ostensibly part time ended up working into their unpaid days as well as their evenings and weekends. Why get paid 75 per cent, she said, when you could be paid 100 per cent for the more than fulltime work that you are probably doing right now? And if you only do 80 per cent work for a 100 per cent salary, think of how many men there are around you doing less for more. She was right. I went fulltime.

Reversals

It was around that time that I had a revelation. There was no longer any reason why I should travel any less than my partner, do any more of the dropping off or picking up at nursery, or do any more than my fair share of the getting this lively and difficult small person ready for bed or encouraging him to eat or, indeed, any of the activities associated with his care. I'd done the pregnancy, the birth, the breastfeeding. The natural, biological female, body work of reproduction was over. Everything else could be shared equally. My partner had exactly the same kind of job and was quite able to step fully into the role of coparent. And unlike some of my female friends, all of them card-carrying feminists, I had no sense of territory to defend; there was no part of that caring work that I was unwilling to cede.

As long as I was part time, there was an expectation that I would be the default person to run home to my son, who was now weaned and able to be fed by anyone. Once I was fulltime, it could be recast as a shared responsibility to drop him off and pick him up from nursery. I'd managed one brief trip abroad and had begun to taste the pleasure that another female colleague alerted me to: the hours to myself, a whole night's uninterrupted sleep, and the possibility of eating a meal in a leisurely enough way to enjoy my food. International travel became a guilty secret. Doing all this called for me to individuate myself. I became *me, myself, I* again. That I was able to carve out a life, and a world, that was utterly and completely mine and in which I could experience the exhilarating joy of aloneness spoke to the intensity of my desire for freedom.

As I slowly reclaimed myself, I began to wallow in a feeling of base selfishness. I was besieged with guilt. The more I enjoyed my freedom, the worse I felt. But it didn't stop me craving my own space, booking more travel, and becoming more and more absorbed in my work. It was some while before I became aware of what had happened. The more I had retreated from the space of responsibility that tends to be occupied and sometimes fiercely defended by women, the more my partner claimed that space as his. And the more he asserted his presence in that space—at first with some rebuke and later with a sense of propriety—the less I was living out a conventional narrative of motherhood.

It was one thing being an equal parent. But ceding the role of primary carer was something entirely different. People would comment on how nice it was that my partner helped, not realizing that I had now become the helper. He was the one to bond with the mums in the playground, the one who bought the presents for the birthday parties our children were invited to, the one to plan their own parties. And there was a strangeness to it. My own uncomfortableness echoed discomfort I sensed in others. I got on better with the dads. We talked about cars, football, work. My partner and I knew no one else who was like this. I came to think of it in terms of role reversal: he'd become the mother and I'd become the father. One of my friends commented that she would find it impossible to fancy a man who did that much of the mothering; he would no longer be masculine enough for her. Caught in a heteronormative frame, all of this—my reaction, their reactions—reinforced my sense of having become other to myself. It did little to help me think past the narrowness of my understanding of what it was to parent and towards a more liberating, feminist way of conceiving of parenting.

Caring Commitments

My work became all absorbing. I had found myself in a leadership role. As fast as I could generate ideas, I spun them into commitments to others. I ended up surrounded by people who could make demands on me and to whom I was endlessly responsive. I spent far too much time at work. I was always on the phone, on email, or in a meeting. I found it exciting, rewarding, and affirming. I had my daughter in the middle of an exhilarating set of projects; my son by then almost five years old. I remember producing a matrix that determined just how much or little involvement would be needed from me for each project during the time I'd be off work. Each piece relinquished felt like a loss. I adored my sparky son and my gorgeous baby daughter. I'd gaze at them amazed to think they'd come out of my body, lark around and play with them as if I were a child, too. My love was passionate, unbridled, unconditional. But work always pulled me back, even when I tried to hold it at bay.

The consequence of all this was that their father moved from sulky critique of my lack of responsibility and presence to fully occupying the space of the primary caregiver. It was for him a role removed from the models offered by his own father and male relatives, even his friends. He remains unique among them. We'd never really discussed what we expected of each other or how we'd parent. But I don't think he intended to find himself in this position. I think he found himself by being placed involuntarily in this position and simply stepped into the vacuum; by vacating the role of primary carer, I like to think I opened the space for him to find a different way of being a father. It has been profoundly affirming for him, bringing him real joy and fulfilment. And for me, inhabiting motherhood from a position of independence has meant I can give myself to it in ways I could not have imagined. From this place,

I love my children and love being their mother all the more.

This feminist mothering of mine has, however, brought with it continual anxious reflection, contradictions, and dilemmas. Stepping back from directing my care into my nuclear family and redirecting it to others brought with it those familiar feelings of guilt. I was besieged with self-blame. This was enthusiastically echoed by my partner's mother, with whom I fought a battle of attrition. She would arrive bearing stews and her own linens, claiming she did so because I was so busy. Her face communicated the intention behind the gesture: I evidently didn't have time for domestic work, wife work. In retaliation, I baked bread, made homemade soups, and even once produced hand-churned butter in a brazen act of faux-domestic defiance. Frictions with the children's father had turned into a cold separateness and from there into living in separate houses, sharing care of the children for half the week each. We'd negotiated a rigidly defined declaration of equality formalized in a three-page document setting out the terms and conditions, which initially included alternating who had three nights and who had four nights a week with the children on an annual basis. I found myself suddenly free for periods of time long enough to rediscover the pleasures of my own company outside work as well as within it.

Family time brought us all together; own-time gave us the freedom to live apart. And the children dutifully trooped between the houses, rebalancing the clothes and detritus associated with mid-week changeovers from time to time. They became teenagers. My son dated the leader of the feminist society at his sixth form college and kept me on my toes. He went off to university. With one teenager left at home, I pondered a demanding university-wide equalities role. My daughter, by then fourteen, pushed me to apply and prepped me for it, composing for me an interview speech about how the university needed to commit to take action on sexual violence and how I was going to help to make it a safer place for women to be themselves, without threat.

I threw myself into the job with feminist activist passion. It consumed me. And it took me away, again, from being there for her at the end of the school day. I'd feel guilty, so guilty, when I'd text to tell her I would be late home because I was in the middle of helping someone else with something that just couldn't wait until tomorrow. Or that I'd be late and then later still because the meeting I was attending spilled over and I just couldn't extract myself. I'd explain it to her when I got home and see a relationship with them, as they grow up and find their own way in the world, as a way of being in which we seek to relate to one another in a way that is as free as possible from societal gender norms, expectations, and obligations. That they regularly reprimand me for any unwitting gender normativity helps us all to stay real.

It is perhaps idealistic to imagine, as I sometimes fondly do, that the intergenerational aspects of parenting could be displaced with an anarchist ethic of nonhierarchical coresponsibility. And I frequently lapse into the tired old ways I imbibed as a child growing up in an era where women like my mother rarely had an opportunity to do anything but endure the life of the house-bound spouse. My son will come home and joke that I must have been trying to meet a deadline, the house is so unnaturally clean. (My mother would do the opposite: spray furniture polish in the air to give the semblance of a day of dutiful housework when she'd actually spent the whole afternoon laughing with her friends.) I bake cakes in efforts to compensate for stretches of absence or for not paying close enough attention to what's going on in their lives. I try and live with adolescent chaos strewn around us all until someone other than me snaps and clears it up; I often fall into living like a teenager myself. But it more than makes up for my shortcomings when my son and I text each other pictures of dishes we've cooked and want to cook for each other, and my daughter and I trade one-liners for dealing with patriarchs at school and at work, even if I can't ever hope to match her best line ever to a teacher who told her off for wearing a skirt that was too short—"why are you looking at my legs, Sir?"

My feminism has made me into a different kind of parent. My son and I chat for hours on the phone. We're still having those philosophical dialogues, picking apart arguments, and exploring the contours of their possibilities. I never ask him if he's eating his vegetables or getting enough sleep. And as my daughter turns sixteen, I contemplate what kind of coming-of-age present might best symbolize that relationship of comrade, friend and mentor. I reflect on my own adolescent sexuality and how long it took me to become the proud owner of my own pleasure. I toy with the idea of the laughter we'd enjoy at the breakfast table on her birthday when she unwraps the present I'd like to buy her—a vibrator, the best model I know of, in glorious bright pink. But then I think: look, she should make her own choices and do things her own way. Let me instead give her gifts that signify and affirm her defining for herself what direction she wants to take next. Isn't that what a feminist parent is good for?

Works Cited

Edholm, Felicity., Olivia Harris, and Kate Young. "Conceptualising Women," *Critique of Anthropology*, vol. 9, no. 10, 1977, pp. 101-30.

Gordon, Tuula. *Feminist Mothers*. New York University Press, 1990.

Horwitz, Erika. "Resistance as a Site of Empowerment: The Journey away from Maternal Sacrifice." *Mother Outlaws: Theories and Practices of Empowered Mothering*, edited by Andrea O'Reilly, Women's Press, 2004, pp. 43-58.

O'Reilly, Andrea. *Mother Outlaws: Theories and Practices of Empowered Mothering*. Women's Press, 2004.

O'Reilly, Andrea. *Feminist Mothering*. SUNY Press, 2008.

Rich, Adrienne. *Of Woman Born: Motherhood as Experience and Institution*. W.W. Norton & Co., 1976.

Chapter 16

Feminist Parenting: No Rock, No Egg!

Toucouleur

It shall not be a fashion statement, a performative "wokeness," a new buzz word, or a simple #hashtag. It cannot be an acquired triumph, a destination, or an award one gets to win. Feminist parenting to me starts before birth, combines both past and present experiences, and continues even after we leave this earth; its ripple effect positively influences the future of boys and girls, men and women. It is a legacy. It is a perpetual scrutiny of the way we think, feel, behave, expect, judge, see, and evolve in our highly gender polarized societies. It is about changing the narratives of boys and girls as well as men and women so that their existence in society is not hampered, reduced, separated, or unfairly treated because of their gender. Feminist parenting entails more than having feminists as parents. It also involves the parenting of actual feminists.

My understanding of the very necessity of feminism as a radiant path to the reclamation of freedom and justice for women and men, boys and girls, all began with how I grew up with my mother within our Senegalese community and how I became conscious of my gender and its consequences within society—and within my inner self. I call this journey my "feminist enlightenment"—a path that keeps widening within and with me, as I have grown from a little girl, to a young woman, and now to a parent who is reflecting upon feminist parenting. Both in my reflections and enlightenment, I have extracted great inspiration and guidance from the nexus of my mother's stories, my existence, and the contexts in which we have both evolved as girls, women, and as mothers.

At an early age, I could see and feel society's gender-based expectations on both my mother and me. Eventually, it felt like we were tangled within the same web of social outlooks: our shared gender was the common denominator. I first saw my mother navigating through those expectations, one step at a time, carefully, diplomatically, in different yet sometimes overlapping functions—as a girl, a young woman, a sister, a daughter, a wife, and a (single) mother. Additionally, we were born Muslims, another important and significant layer added to the blend of gender, religion, culture, space, and situation. Sometimes, depending on the social setting, one role would be more appreciated and/or assessed than the other. Nonetheless, for our gender, it was obvious that submission and utmost respect is always expected, demanded, and applauded at all levels. Our existence as women within the Senegalese society, just as in many settings, has been significantly different from that of boys and men due to a never-fading gender aspect, simply because we were born women.

Feminist parenting means raising my children to understand the foulness within all gender stereotypes, especially within the rhetoric of "be a woman," "men don't cry," "this is not ladylike," or "this is not manly," which are all commonly used (somewhat universally) to remind women and girls of their standing in society and to poison boys and men's thinking and ego with such untruths. In my mother tongue, we frequently use *"Jigeen ju man góor,"*[1] *"waaw-*góor*,"*[2] and *"góor góor lul"*[3] without any frequent analysis of our language. Feminist parenting would question this and what it entails for our boys and girls, who will then become men and women, make up communities, and perpetuate traditions beyond semantics. When in simple expressions of gratitude, encouragement, or praise, parents, extended family, friends, and strangers use heavily gender-charged expressions, what does it do to children's thinking? How will it affect boys' interactions with girls or men's interactions with women? Feminist parenting would ask why we compare boys and girls. At an early age, I could see and feel how my mother internalized and externalized such social stresses, on herself and onto me, either by denouncing them, simply calling them out, or following the rules for some peace of mind. Indeed, some of these pressures can be heavy and can put one person against an entire family, especially against the elders, who are to be revered and respected at all cost.

Parenting in Senegal is mostly about understanding that "the parent is a rock while the child is an egg."[4] As a child (and even as an adult), going against what parents want—even if it is their projection of social gender-based expectations, boundaries, and judgments—would be a disgrace. I was taught as much from what I saw in my family and in many others in Senegal through my mother (the egg) and my grandmother (the rock). Their relationship, or the rock to be specific, has always made me reconsider my night outings in downtown Dakar—wearing short dresses or skirts to reveal my long shea-buttered legs, having male friends over, dressing up like a boy, wearing tight pants, and beyond. My male cousin could do whatever he wanted, unlike me. "He is a boy," I would be told, emphasizing that he was born a boy hence with "more freedom than me." Ironically, the exact words used would always stress the fact that I needed to stay home for safety reasons. Indeed, my late rock-solid grandmother was the social ambassador of our traditions and culture—the matriarch. On many occasions, my nonabiding and not-as-diplomatic-as-my-mother self would challenge her. I watched my mother secretly defend me yet cringe at these egg-breaking circumstances—I had a hard shell, baby!

From the way my mother treated my grandmother with love and respect, although their parenting ideas were opposites, I learned the importance of never completely replacing different perspectives with mine. I also understood that vicinity was important to creating opportunities for dialogue and mutual understanding. Feminist parenting will tell parents and children to not shy away from tough conversations or to push aside their or others' differences. Such a position creates a solid foundation of dialogue on human rights, justice, and equality, empowering diversity in cultures as well as in opinions. Besides, I also saw my mother struggle to please both her daughter and society as well as to reconcile her conflicting parenting choices with other people's approaches. Both my mother and I were constantly being told that women and girls are supposed to behave a certain way. But my mother was not afraid to listen to herself and to secretly give me freedom.

As a single parent with no high school diploma and no financial independence, there were many obstacles to my mother's wellbeing and to my upbringing. She depended on regular family support. Perhaps that dependency made her more vulnerable to egg-breaking judgments regarding everything she did, including her parenting. In contrast, I used to think that perhaps with my financial stability and with having studied abroad for almost a decade and by becoming this so-called emancipated African woman, I could bypass my society's gendered expectations in how I live and parent. But this thought is wrong, as it oversimplifies things; it assumes that financial independence or modernity would systematically create more opportunities and fewer restraints for women. However, feminist parenting will say that women with no jobs, women with no education, women in Senegal, and women everywhere— all women—are deserving of respect and independence, with no conditionality attached.

My mother felt that the key to my freedom was education, both at home and at school. She provided me with a rock solid educational foundation, leading to several academic diplomas and a MasterCard Foundation scholarship to study abroad; I was the first woman in my family to receive an undergraduate degree. But I also know this achievement is my mother's, too. In her eyes, I am a successful woman. However, besides becoming an academic, there is also what the Senegalese society describes as "a successful woman," which includes marriage, motherhood, and appearance,[5] a collective Senegalese disbelief on "*l'habit ne fait pas le moine.*"[6] In a proud way, I see my mother's different approaches (her parenting, her dreams for me, her belief in my potential regardless of my gender, and the way she chose her own definition of a successful woman) key pillars of feminism: freedom, choice, and justice. Feminist parenting will tell parents that girls and boys are blessings. It will simply and equally teach boys and girls that success is reaching your aims in life, being the best version of yourself, and making this world a better place, at your own level.

Deep within, I am so grateful of my mother's stories, her magnificent and powerful step back from social norms, as well as how she tackled thorny sexist boundaries in her own childhood. Feminist parenting should value the sharing of such stories, wound marks, and healings; feminist narratives should recount pain and joy as well as mistakes and accomplishments. My mother's stories are part of my heritage. I treasure them like a library or like an art exhibit I look at for inspiration—a place I visit to ensure past mistakes are fixed in my present and avoided in my children's future, since "those who do not know history are condemned to repeat the same mistakes." Likewise, feminist parenting lets boys and girls visit the past (and the past of each other) to see, hear, touch, and feel with all five senses what it is/was like to be in the other's shoes.

I will tell my children that my mother was the first-born girl. She had the responsibility of cooking, doing the laundry, and cleaning while her brothers were to stay away from such so-called female chores. My mother, like many other girls in the 1960s, did not finish primary school. She would always tell me how terrified she was of her teacher. The male teacher would beat the students who did not behave well or who failed the tests. Her terror continued at home, where one of her older brothers would teach the younger siblings in the same manner the teacher did at school. Don't children repeat what they see? Don't they perpetuate it? Physical punishment has been an integral part of education in many countries, including Senegal. My mother taught me (and those who ever dared touch me) that physical punishment has no place in children's upbringing—not at school, not at home, not anywhere. Her story taught me that violence towards boys and girls, against men and women is simply wrong.

In her child mind, she unfortunately understood that education equated beatings, so she chose not to go to school. She later became beyond determined to send me to school and to make sure I had the right treatment. She taught me to be a super involved parent and to make sure that my children get the best education, in places where no traumatic experiences would interfere with their learning or with their lives. My going to school was her effort to fix past mistakes. She broke a vicious cycle of girls not attending school. Feminist parenting also inspires the breaking of such bad cycles. Since then, she has been an antiviolence advocate. I will tell my children that this shaped my antiviolence activism, which I expressed through performing arts in my high school, promoting the eradication of gender-based obstacles. My mother's parenting included meaningful storytelling. In my feminist parenting, I will use the avenue of storytelling to have a similar positive impact on my boys and girls.

Later on in life, my mother's stories empowered me to leave my abusive marriage—an act that led to me being called a "bad wife," a "bad mother," and an "incomplete woman," since by leaving my husband, I would be "without a man." Her stories told me that the slightest abuse should not be tolerated. Her stories prepared me for tough choices I had to make that put me in front of a hot social glare. During these "hot" moments, I also experienced and questioned marriage and parenting, how they are taught and shown by the Senegalese society, as well as the expected role of the woman, the role of the man, and the two bounded together "until death do us apart." I chose to never put myself or my children in any toxic environment, even if that meant dismantling sacred covenants and living without a man. I am, with or without a man. I am.

Feminist parenting is accountability. It tells me to be honest about these tough life decisions and to not be silent about my truth as my children deserve to know. The truth shall set them free; it will teach them that parents are not perfect human beings and that people should be accountable to their own mistakes. In fact, one thing that suffocated my existence while I was in my abusive marriage was the complete silence and the pretending that everything was okay just to placate society's expectations. Feminist parenting wants, gives, demands, teaches, and passes on the truth; it demands we speak up. Whereas my mother broke the cycle of uneducated girls, I broke the cycle of physical violence. My children shall break more barriers; they will themselves confront the past and learn from it, and they will strive for increased equality and justice for future generations as well. Hence, feminist parenting requires a thorough cleansing, assessment, as well as continual evaluation of so many aspects of our lives. The general tendency is to pass down the good, but the bad too needs to be told, understood, and seen as a source of valuable lessons.

I shall treat my feminist parenting as a form of continuous self-assessment concerning my thought processes, perspectives, judgments, and actions. The issue is not just society and its distortions, the collectively normalized standards, and gender binaries. The issue is also the lies we continue to live with. For a long time I hesitated to leave my marriage for I believed that would make me a "bad mother" as I would be separating my children from their father. Feminist parenting encourages unlearning these lies. It started with me unlearning that girls are inferior to boys. It continues, as I teach my kids that it is okay for boys to cry and provide a definition of marriage that sees both husband and wife as equals. It critiques the rock vs. the egg analogy. Our experiences as children, as well as the guidance of our elders, help us make decisions concerning the legacy we want to leave to our children and to the world. Therefore, feminist parenting must evaluate the legacy we live in and shall one day leave behind. It is not a perfect formula; feminist parenting is feminist parenting in progress. It takes work. It takes both unlearning lies and learning rights. It takes challenging others and challenging the self, a continuous examination. In fact, we must examine our present and revisit our lives as boys and girls as well as men and women in order to evaluate the effect our upbringings have had on our worldviews. What do we see? What do we learn? How do we create better equality and justice through the way we exist and parent our boys and girls? Can we fix past mistakes? Can we erase past ignorance? What do we want to pass down to our children? This is feminist parenting to me—persistent reflection, acknowledgment, correction, deconstruction, questioning, and creation. Such a practice of feminist parenting is required to make our children better informed boys and girls, men and women, as well as more aware and better members of the global community.

I am learning to grasp, detect, condemn, and cleanse myself of social stereotypes regarding gender. I must do this to become freer and happier, to know the importance of humanism and justice, and to enjoy my womanhood, humanity, motherhood, and individuality. We must understand the world and the community we live in, our cultures and religions, as well as their expectations and barriers in order to better grasp how the world affects and influences boys and girls as well as men and women. We need to know how barriers get created and how to deconstruct them. For me, this is the essence of feminist parenting; it is simply cultivating my self-awareness and self-reflection. It is about enlightening myself first and then inviting my children to join our enlightenment journey. As a feminist parent, I will encourage my kids to challenge everyone, including me, to question and fight against the injustices they see around them, whether it be directed to them or to others. Undoubtedly, this will make the world a better place for all.

Endnotes

1. This is an expression to congratulate powerful, successful, and hardworking women, in relation to men. It is a Wolof sentence to accolade or praise but literally means a woman who is more powerful than a man.
2. "*Waw*" means "yes," and "*góor*" means "man" in Wolof. Literally, together "*waaw-góor*" means "yes man," a Wolof expression to say "well done, Brava!"

3. "*Góor góor lul!*" is said to encourage anyone, including girls—for instance, "You better *góor góor lul* for the next exam so you get better scores" or "You are a such a hard worker, keep it up, "góor góor lul!"
4. This is a popular Wolof saying that perfectly paints the parent-child relationship dynamic.
5. Always looking at your best with fancy clothes, especially on social occasions like weddings, family gatherings, and naming ceremonies, is important.
6. This is French for "do not to judge a book by its cover," but literary meaning is that the "clothes do not make a beggar." Here I highlight how the opposite of this belief exists in Senegal, where clothes occupy a significant part of the Senegalese collective understanding regarding success. What one wears becomes a visual marker of his or her success, unsurprisingly more so for women than men.

Chapter 17

Liberating One's Self: Healing and Helping Others Do the Same

Joanna Grace Farmer

I created my company, Building Community Capacity, to focus on increasing access to information and resources that strengthen and empower children, families, and communities. We work at the intersection between education and community development, and share possibilities and opportunities that can help people reach their highest potential. I hope to leave lasting memories of using my ancestral legacy of faith, hope, and love to help create necessary change and increase collective wellbeing, especially for those less fortunate.

My life has been a journey of lifelong learning. Along the way, I've been able to develop expertise in community development, housing, education, parenting, mental health, cultural competency, transformative pedagogy, and evaluation. As an African-American woman, I am blessed to carve out a path so I can help provide equitable access to information and resources that create better life outcomes. To create strategies that result in necessary change, I study and practice cultural relevancy by using Sankofa to reach back and fetch what's necessary to move forwards. I also use the seven principles of the Nguzo Saba and forty-two ideals of the Maat to develop culturally relevant initiatives and programs.

When I was asked to write an essay about feminist parenting, I thought about my ancestors and the women in my family who I watched take on the world. In a patriarchal and hierarchical society—focused on race, gender, class, income, and zip code as well as positioned to establish dominance and oppression—a woman's inherent value can be diminished and denigrated. Unfortunately, the resulting impact on a woman's self-worth can be debilitating. I thought about the women I've been blessed to interact with during my life journey—the ones who have encouraged me to defy persistent stereotypes placed before us through television, movies, magazines, newspapers, and music. Although we lamented during our heartfelt conversations about the state of a world where women could be converted to anything but the human beings divinely equipped to bring life into the world, we also resolved that we would negate society's debilitating images of women by using what we were witnessing to correct these perceptions and stop the behaviour. Feminist parenting is for those willing to defy the status quo while shifting the paradigm to one that increases collective wellbeing.

Perseverance is an asset when you're an African-American woman and determined to maintain your integrity, sanity, and dignity. This chapter is derived from traumatic events and my struggle to successfully manage bipolar disorder, a mental illness. My spiritual beliefs and values of liberation have helped me overcome what seemed impossible. Learning from my relapses meant I had to dig deeper so I could cope with trauma in ways that empowered me to take better care of myself. While in recovery, I used my time to learn more about self-care and which practices would help me be stable, more resilient, and able to thrive. Yes, I struggled while earning degrees in public policy studies and sociology from the University of Chicago as well as in curriculum and instruction from the University of Missouri-Kansas City. I experienced multiple relapses, and I have been blessed to create self-care practices that put me in a better position to be a feminist parent and help those less fortunate.

Unfortunately, tragedy has been a significant feature of my life. From my brother's early passing because of a fall from a third-storey porch to my parents' suicides, I grew used to sometimes unbearable pain. But I have to remember my parents' powerful example of being givers and helpers, whether it was advice, money, or a place to live. They left powerful memories of focusing on family and celebrating milestones. They left a legacy of love and affection that's a model for my feminist parenting. I am blessed to channel their goodness when I work with people who have lost hope and feel unloved. I use my journey of healing to help.

Being a six-year-old girl in a world that limits one's ability to be smart and successful could have been more challenging, but I was blessed with a family that encouraged my brilliance and confirmed my insight and wisdom. Having adults who listened to my ideas about the way things should work was a vital part of my childhood, resulting in a humble pride and an optimistic outlook. I was confident and more secure until my childhood was affected by tragedy in 1968, when Martin Luther King Jr., a hero and force to be reckoned with, was assassinated. I remember the day we heard about Dr. King's assassination because of the chaos I heard outside— the shouting, yelling, and gunshots. My parents didn't go to work, something they never did. My father worked as a presser at a dry cleaner, and my mother was a cashier at a local supermarket. I witnessed the horror, panic, stress, and fear expressed by the adults who cried out in anguish, suffering with the knowledge that our king was gone. They learned that he was murdered in Memphis, Tennessee, where he had travelled to unite with sanitation workers seeking to right wrongs and create equality. What I knew most of all is that I couldn't go to school, which, besides being at home with my family, was my favourite place because of my thirst for learning. My family explained that I would have to miss school for a while and wait until things calmed down. Although I loved the extra time and attention I received from my parents, it was a time of emotional and mental challenges as well as of heightened anxiety and fear. Painful memories created issues larger than a six-year-old's ability to process current events. My parents did their best and continued to nurture my appetite for learning; they used a curriculum of their making to reinforce positive and constructive African-American identity and representation.

In my six-year-old version of patience, the schools finally reopened, and I went back to school. Everything had changed. I walked past buildings destroyed and with embers still glowing of fires used to torch them. I wondered why and asked questions of my parents. I learned about racism and the unique form of evil that created structural and institutional inequality and inequity. Mama and Daddy explained that we had a place in American society on the bottom steps of a ladder specifically designed to oppress and keep us there. However, my parents also explained that we did not belong in that place because, as children of The Creator, it was never meant for us to be there. Leading by example, they taught me to defy racist ideology by maintaining a standard of excellence.

harmful side effects of major depression and psychotropic medications.

Mama gave me a journal when I was six years old. It was white with a zipper. It had a tiny lock and key. She encouraged me to write about my dreams. That gift of writing has saved my life because I would write for hours sometimes, putting my secrets on paper—the things I couldn't tell others. My trauma and pain were locked inside me. Journaling was a way to heal and survive as best I could. Mama nurtured my creativity and independence by providing opportunities for me to explore ideas. One year, she gave me a chemistry set; another year, it was a pottery wheel. I would spend hours experimenting with a new formula or design. Having this time helped me with the pain of my trauma, even if only for a little while. I learned to use my time and energy to craft the goals I wanted to achieve so I was free to read, write, create, run, and play. I excelled in school and benefited from the emotional support of my tight-knit family.

Most of our family gatherings were at our three-storey apartment building. My father was known for his love of barbeque, and nothing pleased him more than showing off his skills for smoking meat. He grilled it for hours until it was so tender that the meat fell off the bones. My mother's potato salad and coleslaw were perfect side dishes. Our feasts included freshly squeezed lemonade, sweet potato pies, and coconut cake. My mother also made sure we had vegetables and would make huge salads, corn on the cob, and greens. We laughed and talked while enjoying our food. After eating and cleaning up, we enjoyed card games, television, and telling tall tales. Being with family was perfect, but there was that hole in my heart that only Little Eddie could fill. I knew my baby brother was in heaven, never too far away, and I soothed myself by making him my guardian angel.

I remember seeing a magazine with Africa on the front cover and I asked my parents if I could read it. They enthusiastically responded yes and handed it to me with care. I understood that I should do the same and carefully turned the pages. I wanted to know more about Africa and while reading I asked my parents, "What's an anthropologist? What's an archaeologist?" My parents were happy to define both words, and after hearing them, I proudly proclaimed, "I'm going to Africa one day!" My parents smiled, pleased with my statement. That dream was planted when my parents affirmed, "Joanna Grace, you can do anything you want. There are no limits for the good you can do and the places you will go!" The magazine was *National Geographic,* and I received a copy of it carefully wrapped in brown paper addressed to Ms. Joanna Grace Farmer care of Mr. Edward Farmer. I eagerly awaited my monthly insight into the world of wonders known as Mother Nature. I was nine years old, and this magazine diverted my attention from my grief.

I attended elementary school in Oak Park and travelled to the northwest side of Chicago to attend high school at St. Gregory the Great. It was a wonderful opportunity because the school had the first Teaching English as a Second Language program in the Catholic school system. It was a blessing to interact with international students and make new friends. I was prepared to learn about other cultures and ways of thinking because my elementary school, St. Catherine of Siena, was the same. I was also exposed to other religious faiths and traditions and learned to respect the many pathways to The Creator. I thrived in these environments because diversity was stimulating for me. I didn't like being bored with sameness.

I completed high school and college while navigating prejudice, stereotypes, bigotry, and stigma. One day, I went to my high school locker to get study materials for my next class, and as I approached it, my eyes widened with shock. Big black lettering forming the word "nigger" was hastily sprawled across the front. Some white students had gathered to see what I would do and if I would react. The black students were noisily saying that this wasn't fair and demanded, "Who did this?" The noise attracted the attention of our English teacher who looked around and saw the n-word on my locker. After shooing the students away, he asked me to have a seat in his classroom and told me to wait until he came back. When he returned, he asked me to go to my next class. As I walked towards the door, he thanked me for how I had handled the situation. I looked outside and saw one of our biggest students holding a bucket of water. The white students looked aghast, and the black students were surprised at the fact that this burly and intimidating student was using a brillo pad to scrub my locker. Our English teacher stepped outside the door frame and reminded us all that it was time to go to class. That student never returned to our school.

I learned another valuable lesson while attending high school. I received my first and only F on a paper I wrote about Crispus Attucks, the first man to die in the Revolutionary War. I had a set of black history encyclopedia and copied a beautiful colour picture of Attucks on onion skin paper. My godmother had given me an electric typewriter for my birthday, and I proudly transferred my handwritten notes to my final edition. I submitted the paper the next day and was shocked to see a big red F on the cover page when it was returned. Children weren't allowed to question teachers about mistakes, so I told my mother who told my father. My father rode the bus and L with me the next morning. When we arrived at my school, he told me to go to class and said he would call for me later.

My father discussed the situation with the principal and then asked to include the history teacher. By the time I was summoned to the office, my teacher looked upset and afraid. My father ended the meeting by reminding the principal that he paid my tuition, and it was an investment in my education. He went on to state that he expected teachers to know all history, not just the Caucasian version. I remember students who were passing in the hallway as the bell rang, which was the signal to head to our next class. They stared at my father, who, with his head held high, let me walk him to the front door of the school. He hugged me and reminded me to be good. He never said goodbye. He always said that—"Be good." My father was preparing me for the times I would need to resolve issues at my children's schools. This skill was useful when I helped other parents fight for their children's rights.

When I think about my precious two children, I remember when my son Jonathan was born. Holding him in my arms and marvelling at this boy of mine, I understood what it would mean to lose a child. It was unimaginable, and that's when I knew that my mother was so strong: she had defied the odds by successfully raising three children to adulthood. She lived long enough to welcome her five grandchildren so she could pass on her legacy of faith, hope, and love. It is from my mother that I learned the power and importance of focusing on the now. She would tell me to have fun and enjoy life. You only get one, she'd say. When I was worried, her response was "Just take it to the altar, talk it over with God, and leave the problem there. Your job is to keep putting one foot in front of the other." When I questioned my direction in life, she'd tell me to follow my heart, listen to my intuition, and be true to myself. My mother's wisdom has carried me through many a sleepless night when I had to make difficult decisions.

She was a woman of peace, and my father loved a good debate. He also liked to argue. Her way was to carefully listen and then respond.

My father could become chauvinistic, trying to have the last word. He said mean and hurtful things—words he couldn't take back because he blamed my mother for Little Eddie's death. My mother turned inwards, and I watched her reject my father. My father's arguing and blaming became his downfall because she wouldn't speak to him for days. She also wouldn't cook or express joy in his presence. While he suffered, she taught him about treating her with unconditional respect, not just when he wanted to. There were no ands, ifs, and buts for her. Her example stuck with me because if I had to deal with relationship issues, I exercised the same power and taught men to respect me as a woman and mother. Mama's behaviour was a lesson in feminist parenting because she didn't subscribe to status quo views of marriage. She knew about the Black Madonna and African beliefs in which women were held in high esteem.

My mother's way of relating to my father was a model for my growing independent way of thinking and behaving. Whereas my father's skilful arguing had increased my critical thinking ability, my mother's commitment to being different helped me do the same. Like her, I refused to conform to stereotypes. My second brother Adam is twelve years younger than me, and I remember taking him out for a while to get some fresh air. As he happily looked around and communicated with me in baby talk, an older white woman from our church was walking down the street. I didn't show my shock when she asked if Adam was my baby. Instead, I calmly turned towards her and said, "Mrs. Such and Such, you know this is my baby brother. His baptism was announced in the church bulletin and you congratulated my parents. My mother was holding him when you came over. You also know that I'm in elementary school." She feigned insult, and when she told my parents about how I had, as she said, sassed her, my mother looked her straight in the eye and said, "You offended my daughter." I always admired how my parents stood up to white people.

Although I learned to cope with tragedy, I was dysfunctional and used busyness as a bandage to cover my grief. I didn't know how to grieve. I learned about the five stages of grief, but mine were erratic. My cycles of mania flowed into depression, which was like being in a hole where there's no light to help you find your way out. I lost days and weeks, sometimes months, in my darkness. Medication can be used to alter your mood, but the wrong ones can be fatal. I had confrontations with psychiatrists because the medication dosages they prescribed were greater than my biological ability to metabolize them. I had to make sure my organs weren't damaged beyond repair. Unfortunately, doctors predicted failure more often than my ability to be successful. They also denied more culturally competent mental healthcare because of a racist ideology.

When my son was born in 1983, I was happily pregnant. There was a blizzard the day I went into labour, and once I arrived at the hospital, my doctor was there. We had agreed that I would use an African tradition of birthing, and I sat on an incline instead of lying flat on my back. When Jonathan arrived, the doctor placed him into my joyful arms, and while oohing and aahing over the shape of his head as well as tenderly touching his face, fingers, and toes, he moved towards my breast. I sang the lullabies my mother taught me as he peacefully nursed. I was pleased with his chocolate brown skin but knew that for the rest of his life, until he could do it for himself, I would have to protect and shield him from the damage that racism creates. I knew there would be barriers put in his way to limit access to opportunities, but his genius was undeniable, and my son excelled on multiple levels. He was well liked in school. He had a village that adored him. Jonathan's name means "given by God" and is a variation of my name, which means the same. He is my gift, as he chose me for his mother. It's a sacred responsibility when you bring life to earth, so I have been diligent in the role I'm entrusted to fulfil.

I learned to have unconditional faith after finding out I was pregnant with my daughter Faith in 1991. I immediately stopped taking psychotropic medications that could have harmed her. It put me at higher risk for a relapse, so I was fortunate to have a doctor who prescribed bed rest and weekly group meetings at Emotions Anonymous. We monitored Faith's development using ultrasounds, and the day she was born was filled with tears of joy. She had no birth defects and received a perfect score of ten. As her obstetrician happily put it, she was glowing. Faith got her name because I was worrying one day, praying, and asking The Creator to make sure she was healthy. In response, I heard, "Have faith." That was the first time she stirred in my womb.

I'm blessed to have a daughter who's sensitive like me. She helps me grow and mature as a mother who also needs to be a good role model and mentor. Faith could have inherited the bipolar gene, so I learned while teaching her ways to calm herself. She loved art, and I made sure she had plenty of crayons and paints. Faith would spend hours, just like I did, creating, except she drew elaborate designs on the sidewalk. Both of my children have helped me understand what it means to be and stay healthy. We enjoy going on adventures and making good memories. We have so many pictures! Now that Jonathan and Faith are adults, the tables have turned, and I am blessed with amazing surprises and family time. I learn a lot from them and treasure their school projects and handmade gifts, which are placed on mantles, tables, and shelves. When I look at them, I pause and take a deep breath while saying a prayer of gratitude.

I've been able to use my tragedies as fuel in my work for social, economic, and political justice. My tragedies have prepared me to understand what it means to have righteous indignation, and I raised Jonathan, now thirty-seven years old and happily married to Rasha, and Faith, who's twenty-eight years old and enjoying the work she's doing, to have the same. They're making excellent choices on their journey called life, and I admire their compassion for others and commitment to justice. Yes, they've been privileged and have benefited from a safe, healthy, happy, and nurturing childhood, but what they've taught me is how all children should have the same. They help me see how living in a world of abundant resources with systems that promote scarcity, individualism, competition, and survival of the fittest is unsustainable. They have an uncanny ability to listen closely while sharing their wisdom and insight about structural racism and the way systems are maintained to deny humans their basic rights for water, food, clothing, shelter, education, and employment. Feminist parents must create the balance and order we need, using strategies based on justice and equity. We have the kind of compassion that helps us see a bigger picture. We must listen closely to what those less fortunate tell us. Their willingness to share their hopes, dreams, and visions for a better world—one with less suffering due to oppression—is part of understanding what it will take to create the change we need. My tragedies inspired me to be a clarion voice for the health, safety, and wellbeing of children, families, and communities. I stand firm in my calling as an organizer and scholar-activist, which is a solid foundation for feminist parenting.

Our ancestors, while enduring the oppression they faced, were clear. They wanted better for their descendants, including access to opportunities. We are still fighting oppression in 2018— the year we're commemorating the assassination of a man not yet forty years old. His

Chapter 18

"Just Wait until They Go to School": Autonomy, Identity, and Feminist Parenting in an Imperfect Society

Danya Long

Perhaps the ultimate lesson of parenthood is one that transcends all cultural, political, and philosophical boundaries: our children refuse to conform to our expectations. Through their insistence on being and becoming their own person, our children lead us through the humbling, joyous, relentless journey of parenthood.

I conceived my first child—deliberately, stubbornly, ambitiously—as a single mother, a lesbian single mother, no less, in a family that already contained many more women than men. Although I had mentally explored the prospect of having a male child—after all, the probability of this was fractionally over one-half—I had never seriously envisaged myself with a son. The baby I remembered most strongly was my sister, and, unconsciously, this was largely what I expected of a baby: averagely sized, averagely gestated, averagely possessing of ten fingers and ten toes, a girl.

He was a boy. "I am thankful that one of my children is male, since that helps to keep me honest" (78) writes Audre Lorde—a provocative assertion and one that resonates for me time and again. I no longer have the luxury of being able to indulge in easy solutions to problems of sexism in action, to sex discrimination, to rape culture, and to male violence. There is a particular complexity to raising a boy child as a feminist—not necessarily more difficult than raising a girl child but certainly more complicated. This baby's maleness sent me back to the drawing board often; my instincts did not always suffice and required second, third, fourth, and fifth guessing. With an imagined daughter, I had an immediate kinship. Almost without thinking, I knew how to foster her strength, self-worth, intellect, and independence; I knew how to celebrate the female form and female achievements, how to role-model a refusal to conform. It was not that I thought this imaginary young woman's existence would be identical to mine, but that (I expected) there would be a great deal of common ground to start from. It was not only this common ground between us either: a society that assumes that maleness is both the default and the preferable option is far more understanding of girls (if not women) who gravitate towards masculine markers and refuse to stay in their box. Tomboys are almost always tolerated and often much admired; "strong women" are respected, as long as they do not seek to be defined beyond the "strong *for a woman*" restriction. Teaching my imaginary daughter to be strong without restriction and to refuse to accept being diminished sounded demanding, but at least I could articulate the aim to myself. But what was I to teach my son? What were the attributes I would need to equip him with to counteract the wider British culture that would tell him he was to be strong, unemotional, important, and powerful? How best should I retain those messages that I would wish a child of any gender to grow up with—that is, that you can do anything you want to do—without unwittingly exacerbating the societal problems patriarchy engenders? How do you help a young man to grow up to be part of the solution, without inducing guilt or risking resentment?

Before I had started trying to conceive, when the hopes, fears, yearning, and magic of imagined motherhood swirled through my mind, a thought I frequently returned to was the prospect of having a son. My desire for a baby had predated my desire for a child, and so too my desire for a daughter predated my desire for a child of unspecified gender. I waited until I was comfortably reconciled to that possibility before beginning my journey. I remember sitting alone one afternoon, college textbooks beside me on a bench in a park near my workplace; I watched a small toddler boy amble along beside his father, pausing at length in serious contemplation of the gravel path. He crouched to pick up a single small stone, held it almost reverently between his forefinger and thumb as he considered it; with precision and great attention, he then dropped it back to the ground and squatted to pick up another. After dropping a number of pebbles, each no less carefully than the first, he took his father's hand again; his curiosity was evidently sated. I watched the boy, and I liked him. I sent a text message to my mother, flippant but truthful: "Very sweet boy-child in the park. I might be happy to have one of those after all."

My instinctive reluctance was not, of course, that I thought male children were really any less sweet than their female counterparts. It was darker and murkier than that. It was the fear that a lone female parent would not be sufficient for a male child and that I would fail my child through my refusal to provide him with a father. It was a hundred newspaper interviews, a thousand flurried camera shots on the steps of some courthouse, where behind some violent criminal— innocent or guilty, apologetic or defiant—stood his mother, eternally responsible, eternally forgiving, somehow complicit when until now I had believed my own femaleness exempted me from complicity. I had a lingering suspicion, frequently shored up by reality,[1] that bringing another man into the world was a reckless thing to do. It was the silly but important question of what to do with him in swimming pool changing rooms and shopping centre toilets. It was the heavy responsibility of bringing up a male child in a culture that too often and too easily directs our male children towards a celebration of violence, and doing so without any first-hand knowledge of how it feels to be a boy and taught this, or how it feels to be male and resist such a lesson.

Parenthood frequently requires us to take a position of great certainty—and one that has a tangible impact—when really we have little clue. I am not a naturally decisive person; for me, feeling perhaps 50 per cent certain about any philosophical or moral position is about as sure as it gets. This equivalence is perfectly adequate to spin out a pub conversation or a seminar discussion; it has served me well in essay writing and in policy analysis, where even a firm conclusion is invariably nuanced. It wins no points as a mother: there is no philosophical 50 per cent in whether a child is vaccinated, how it is fed, where it sleeps, how it is educated, or what family rules and routines it is expected to follow. How I am raising my son as a boy in a feminist household in a patriarchal society has meant a similar series of stab-in-the-dark decisions, backed up by what may pass for evidence, but ultimately led by my gut. To put it more succinctly: for better or worse, we just have to get on with it.

Resisting Gender Stereotypes: Baby Steps

The insidiousness of gender stereotyping is a startling revelation to many parents. The tale is a familiar one; it often begins in a toy shop, where the small plastic kitchens are inexplicably pink, or in a clothing store, where sparkles and practicality are strictly segregated—the one side of the shop targeted at aspiring superheroes and 'rascals' with truck motifs and boisterous slogans ("Here comes trouble!"), the other at the "pretty cute" appreciator of sequins and baby animals. "Toys are for everyone," we say firmly, an argument we did not expect to find still required. We ensure a careful balance in our own homes where dolls and their paraphernalia nestle beside vehicles and train tracks, where the gaudy jewels of the dressing-up box spill over onto the box of building blocks, where the scooter is orange and the buggy is purple because the other available options seemed the equivalent of carrying a neon sign declaring the child's sex. We change the sex of the characters in picture books and wonder why all the animals in *Dear Zoo* are male; we think it is no wonder that boys are widely seen to lack interest in female protagonists when they barely get to meet one. And in twenty-first-century Britain, where the law recognizes how little difference a person's sex makes to their interests and their possibilities, where the notion of certain jobs or rights or pastimes being reserved to only one sex or the other looks like a relic of history, it is jarring to see the explicit gendered message children receive almost from the moment they leave the womb. Women are expected to participate as equals in the workplace, yet girl children are disproportionately encouraged to play at home-making, care-taking, and prettifying themselves: modern childhood, in gender terms, seems inexplicably fifty years out of date.

The extraordinary emphasis on gender begins at birth, if not earlier, given the possibilities of ultrasound. "Girl or boy?" strangers in the street ask, as they stop to smile at my baby. Perhaps there is little else to be discussed about someone so small. It surprises me, in those early months, to contrast the fascinating minutiae of daily life as my baby grows into a person and I grow into a mother, with just how uninspiring the small-talk at the bus stop or the supermarket checkout is: sex, age, sleep, and convenience ("is he good?"). Perhaps we lack the language for the wonder of it all, or perhaps such an outpouring is at odds with British reserve. Despite such banal interactions, through pregnancy and motherhood I feel myself welcomed into an unspoken female collective, able to instantly gain camaraderie and social acceptance simply by identifying myself as a mother. I have friends without children who feel themselves ostracized by this same force; I feel guiltily complicit. What feminism ends up meaning to me, as a mother, becomes far more simplistic and reactive than I had expected: it becomes a feminism primarily about challenging the antifeminism I see around my children. It is the rejection of "girl things versus boy things," whether the things in question are toys or personal attributes or roles in society. It is the refusal to enable male aggression and violence under the guise of "boys will be boys," which is perpetuated in so much of the television and film aimed at boys. It is challenging the assumption that the default is male. It often looks tokenistic, but to children who are forming an understanding of the world based on what they witness every day, these tokens are important.

The Boy in an Elsa Dress

When my son is sixteen months old, I start my MSc program, and he starts nursery. Where I had once been his world, he now has a whole world beyond me: new foods, new songs, new routines, and new companions. Somewhere among the big wooden building blocks, the sandpit, and the strawberries in the garden, he learns to sing "Let It Go." Thus, he knows *Frozen* long before he has ever watched it. Eventually, we watch it. We watch it several times; at some point, it begins to feel that we may have watched it several hundred times. *Frozen* becomes a safe bet for t-shirts and birthday presents. In common with many of his peers, the years aged three to five are easily remembered as "the *Frozen* years." Naïvely, the small boy in an Elsa dress can be regarded as a triumph of gender nonconforming parenting; it is unexceptional (although there is no other such boy in my son's nursery), but it is also a clear signal that this boy has been free to choose and that he has learned to scorn anyone who dares tell him this is not for boys. At the same time, mothers of older children raise an eyebrow. "Just wait until he goes to school," they say. I think I begin to recognize the shift to which they are alluding, as with each passing year the number of his male peers with long hair grows fewer: the children grow incrementally older and are incrementally made more masculine. Gender performance can be deferred, perhaps, but not indefinitely.

the price he is willing to pay rather than adjust himself to fit in with less explanation. If it were not his own choice to do so and be so, I am sure I would still delight in precisely who he was. But I am tremendously grateful he has embraced a way of being that enables him to repeatedly challenge the limitations we impose on boyhood because I believe that in so doing, he continues to nurture an early feeling of pro-feminism in himself and, at least sometimes, provokes reflection in others.

We do not live in a feminist enclave filled with children pushing at the same barriers as he is. When he is nearly six years old, he comes home from the childminders one day, excited by a new playmate who is "another boy who looks like a girl!" He says, "I thought I was the only one in London!" It is the first time that I have heard him refer to himself so explicitly in these terms. His sense of camaraderie and relief is palpable. The geography of his phrase "in London" is slightly off; rather, he is distinguishing our local community from the children of my friends. I feel honoured by this insight and quietly proud that he so happily identifies himself in this way. He knows he is a boy, he knows people perceive him as looking like a girl, and he does not care. He does not sound like a child who has been forced into becoming a suitable accessory for my own politics.

To the question of evangelizing (through) our children, I suspect this is an inevitable feature of parenthood. We impose our own values and norms on our children—explicitly or implicitly—in line with a majority viewpoint or at odds with it. It would have been no less political to have dressed him in the typical dreary browns and blues of boyhood. Indeed, to cultivate a vacuum of neutrality seems absurd. Whether our children end up embracing our values or setting themselves in opposition to what they consider our misguided beliefs, surely we want to raise people who have a positive and passionate contribution to make. It is my hope that my children will lead thoughtful and reflective lives and that they will find fulfillment not only in uncomplicated pleasure but also in challenges, frustration, and hard work.

I do not want to protect my child from realizing that gender is political. Nor do I want to find an oasis of feminism within which to raise him. If such a community exists, it is outside of my knowledge and likely also my budget—not to mention my cultural capital. My son socializes widely and chooses his own friends; I have no power at all over his acquaintances. His playmates cannot be handpicked for having (parents with) a worldview that is compatible with mine. I begin to learn the art of small talk. Parenthood flings me into social situations with a far more diverse range of contacts than any professional or academic setting has done, maybe since my own school days. Or perhaps it's not that exactly—maybe there is no real increase in the diversity of experiences and worldviews, but that a greater degree of friendly interaction is required and that a more personal and more political subject (i.e., our children) is always close at hand, making for a peculiarly honest form of networking.

The media peddles a myth of "mommy wars" between those who breastfeed or use formula or between those who are employed or stay at home with their children. But all these divisions do not translate to my own experience. I do not find that mothers (always mothers!) are as defensive, judgmental, or easily offended as this myth implies. I find myself, and my donor-conceived princess boy, sometimes a curiosity but never an enemy. In conversation with a parent from school, I learn that she thinks I have two children of similar age, one girl and one boy: both of these children, I realize, are, in fact, my son.

"A Rich Man's Family"

When my son is five years old, I conceive my second child, a daughter. "A rich man's family!" remarks a cheerful midwife, as she charts my growing abdomen with her tape measure. The term is new to me: a son to inherit my wealth, a daughter to forge a strategic alliance through marriage. I am reminded of a previous conversation with my son about inheritance. Some months earlier, we tramped through boggy mud at Knole, and talked about Vita Sackville-West and about how tragic it must have felt to so deeply love the home and countryside she had grown up in, and know that but for the randomness of her sex, it would all have been hers. My son shared my response to the landscape and the injustice, with the added bewilderment of a child in twenty-first-century Britain who has no frame of reference for these trappings of patriarchy, who does not realize that the Succession to the Crown Act is younger than he is, and who simply cannot believe that any law could be so ridiculous as to insist that inheritance is a strictly male business. It took him some moments longer to properly grasp the implication for his own family and for himself as the eldest son. The cogs whirred visibly in his brain as he tried to understand my own economic impossibility within that society, a part of history that still seemed in touching distance even to my child as we threw rain-swollen sticks onto the ground to watch them snap, the big house in the distance still inhabited, the tale still very much alive.

In the clinic with the well-meaning midwife who meant only to make friendly conversation, I am economically impossible once more. I share none of these thoughts. The midwife struggles to stretch to an impossible tension the treasury tag connecting my maternity notes, apologizes, and then suggests I ask my husband to do it. I nod and smile. She is warm and pleasant. In this brief appointment, I have concluded I wouldn't mind if she ended up attending me in labour – a clinical success, no matter the implications of her unserious words. Not for the first time, I contemplate this important new business of raising a daughter. I wonder what this daughter raising task will look like and contemplate it more seriously now than when I had dismissed it as conceptually easier for a feminist than raising a son.

My son is unenthusiastic about the news of a forthcoming sibling and more unenthusiastic still when an antenatal scan shows that this sibling will be a sister. Why does he wish for a boy? I wonder. Is it because being a boy is of great import to him? Is it because he feels outnumbered in our family, either as it is already or in the future, when this interloper shares something with me that he does not? Or is it simply one of those random preferences he has declared one day, careless words that become important only to avoid losing face? I cannot tell.

We sort through his old baby clothes, and in flashes, he warms slightly to the whole enterprise; he secretly enjoys hearing tales of his own babyhood as I take out each sleepsuit and remember him by them. Here and there, he removes an item from the pile and insists it is "not for girls." There is no rhyme or reason to what clothing is decreed thus. My belly grows bigger, and his ambivalence grows stronger. In the supermarket, he spontaneously selects a sleepsuit from the sale rail. My concern is his adjustment to big brotherhood, and I do not query his selection—that he wants to help dress a baby he has been so painfully opposed to is positive. He has chosen a pink sleepsuit with a sewn-in tutu and a Disney princess motif. Weeks later, his sister wears it when she is not yet a whole day old. I wonder what on earth prompted his choice, whether it is his own gender-unrestricted liking for it or his gender-restricting prescription for a girl baby, or perhaps the one disguised by the other. There is no way on earth my daughter would have ever worn such a thing, if she had not been preceded by a brother; I wonder what that means, too. Probably it is little more than lazy signalling on my part. I cringe when the midwife comes to check on us both the day after the birth and the baby is wearing this garish monstrosity. The midwife is interested in feeding, jaundice, meconium, and lochia; the politics of the baby's outfit are unlikely to register.

My daughter is born with one hand up beside her head. "Like a superhero," I tell my son, who has been working on a "heroes" topic at school. "Marxist salute," says my mother. "Black power," I reply. I buy her a Superman outfit because the coded reference to her compound birth presentation pleases me. I am not sure whether I would have bought it for a boy child. We are back to the tokenism of clothing. Still, the tokenism remains inescapable because it remains relevant: the nurse assumes she is a boy when she wears the Superman outfit to her first set of vaccinations and encourages my son to "tell him he's a good boy" as she wails in pain. When I smile and say, "Actually, she's a good girl," the nurse apologizes, and tells me my daughter has the face of a girl and the sleepsuit of a boy. "Ah, but you saved it from him?" she says, indicating my son. I wonder what sort of success rate anyone might have by guessing a baby's sex from face alone. I remember how often people apologized for thinking my son female by saying it was because he was so beautiful. Truthfully, guessing "she" when faced with my baby son in a bright floral t-shirt was statistically a sensible thing, but people rarely blamed my clothing choices, politely shoring up the notion of intrinsically-beautiful-but-diminishing femininity instead—"I'm sorry. Your son only looks like a girl because he is so beautiful. I'm sorry. Your daughter does look like a girl. I only thought she was a boy because she is dressed in blue."

I wonder who my daughter will grow up to be and whether she will insist on her right to be who she is as fiercely as her brother has.

The Quiet Feminism of Being

In the end, children learn from what they experience rather than what they are told. To marry a few themes together, we might say that feminist parenting is about "deeds, not words." I had not anticipated that so much of family life would be taken up with challenging casual sexism, or that gendered expectations would be lurking around every corner. I had not expected so much energy to be taken up in defending a boy's right to do girl things. I hope I am doing nothing so narrow and regressive. Rather, I hope that by helping to expand the breadth of what a boy and a man can be, my son and I are contributing to a net reduction in toxic masculinity. We will not win any prizes for radical action, but I believe our daily visible resistance of antifeminism remains a valuable contribution. I am proud of my son's refusal to conform, even when he felt that he was "the only one in London"; I hope he will always have the courage and integrity to stand alone and unapologetic when circumstances demand it.

I perceive that the very act of my parenthood—specifically, my choice to go it alone—to be a feminist one; it is not the only feminist option but certainly a valid one that I do not regret. I wonder whether the message I think my son has internalized, and which my daughter will too in time—that mommy does it all—is as positive as I hope it is. If a conventional heterosexual couple form the first impression for their children's understanding of relationships as well as family and gender roles, what conclusions are my children guided towards? I hope I have shown them and others that alternative family configurations are possible and positive. I hope my children of both sexes will be loved and supported, emotionally and practically, by those they choose to have around them, but I also hope that they will have the capability and the courage to be self-sufficient when their circumstances or preferences demand it. For both children, above all, I hope that they will not feel they have been hard done by through the circumstances of their birth. I hope neither feels unduly constrained by their sex, and I hope both will (continue to) grow up to challenge shoddy thinking, and its human costs, wherever they find it.

Endnotes

1. For example, 78 per cent of perpetrators of violent crime in England and Wales are male (Office for National Statistics).

Works Cited

Lorde, Audre. *Sister Outsider: Essays and Speeches.* Crossing Press, 1984.

Office for National Statistics. "The Nature of Violent Crime in England and Wales: Year Ending March 2017." *ONS*, www.ons.gov.uk/peoplepopulationandcommunity/crimeandjustice/articles/the nature ofviolentcrimeinenglandandwales/yearendingmarch2017 #what-do-we-know-about-perpetrators-of-violent-crimes). Accessed 14 Feb. 2020.

Chapter 19

Sidestepping the Patriarchy: Creating in Our Children a Critical Feminist Consciousness

Sehin Teferra

Introduction

I am a professional feminist. I am the co-founder and coordinator of one of the first feminist networks in Ethiopia, and have a PhD in gender studies. So, one would think that when I became a parent, which I had desperately wished to be, I would have naturally taken the feminist route. However, there were factors at play deeper and older than feminism, and I ended up taking a longer road to feminist parenting.

In time, I found that my eight-year-old daughter Rekka, and my five-year-old son Leeben are more significant than the nonegalitarian marriage that their father and I were in and that I had to leave it in order to find my way to a more authentic feminist parenting, in which, in the words of Chimamanda Ngozi Adichie, I matter equally. In this chapter, I reflect on the journey of consciously parenting along feminist principles. I share what that means for my feminist goals of raising children who value justice and equality while doing it as a single parent.

Parenting is daunting, and feminist parenting requires vigilance. I want to teach my daughter the lessons I learned the hard way—that being a feminist starts with self-love and to not settle for friends or lovers who do not see her worth. Parenting a boy, in contrast, has led me to a deeper questioning of my values as well as to an exploration of the complex trappings of the man box, which I try to keep my son out of; I teach him to not stand in the way of women. My reflections in this chapter represent an outline of a critical path I am learning to lead my children on in the pursuit of a more just future.

I was recently speaking to a leading Ethiopian feminist activist who has parented two remarkable women and who is now a grandmother to two boys and one girl. She was taken aback when I said that in Ethiopia, becoming a man is as difficult as becoming a woman, but she heard out my explanations. The more I learn from parenting my daughter and son, the more that I have come to believe that the path of parenting children of either gender requires precision and a vast amount of the purest love that you can access. I agree that the task of raising a girl who will become a woman in this unequal world is daunting, but I am also of the opinion that raising a boy needs an equal conscientious effort. The notion that boys will get by because they are naturally tougher has put many men in vulnerable positions, in which they feel underloved and undernurtured in a society that encourages them to act out in aggressive ways. It is similar to being put on a precipice that requires careful negotiation to descend while the crowds on the ground are encouraging you to jump.

Raise Them the Same but Not the Same

I think it's great when women and men say that their parents always treated them the same as their siblings of another gender. If we teach our sons to bake and cook without making it a big deal, we are equipping them to feed themselves and not to simply help their future wives, assuming they will get married. If you encourage your daughter to be physically active and to rely on herself, she will grow up to be a self-assured woman. This I believe is Feminist Parenting 101, but let's not end there.

I think that as feminist mothers, we need to teach our girls to be self-confident, for sure, but also to uplift other women. We should tell our daughters to steer clear of men who are threatened by their ambition but also to make sure that they think beyond their own gains. We should teach them to be kind to everyone but to express particular solidarity with girls who may not have it as easy as they do. We should encourage them to stand up for themselves, for sure, but also to support the girl in the class who is teased about her weight or her unconventional looks. They should be aware of injustice, but particularly gendered injustice. Such an approach takes practice, but what has worked for me in developing my daughter's sensibility around gender is to follow a strict rule in my interaction with other women. I plan to call her out on any catty remarks she might make about classmates or friends, as unlikely as that scenario seems now. Her current best friend is a boy, but she has other close friends who are girls. In her short tenure at kindergarten, we have already had the difficult task of negotiating a case of bullying by another girl which required much feminist handwringing on my part. I wanted to use the opportunity to teach her to stand up for herself without falling into the dangerous "girls are like that" trap, which has set many women of my generation up for unnecessary angst.

At the end, my daughter ended up delivering her much-rehearsed "I will not play with you anymore, as you have been mean to me several times" line and that was the end of that— for now. I am sure there will be more people like that in my children's lives and they will be boys and girls. There may even be a time when it is my child who is in the guilty seat. My feminist take on the unfortunate reality of bullying is to emphasize that it is not the natural domain of femaleness, even though it is what society and popular media would have us believe.

Am I saying that women and girls are not often cruel to each other in quite specific feminine ways? I wish I could argue that, but we all know better, as there are women who eye you with aggression the minute you walk into a room and who make nasty judgments before they get to know what you are about. When my male friends observe that women are not nice to each other, I wish I could honestly say that has not been my experience, but I can't. What I can and do say is that I see through it. I see through the unnecessary competition that is bred from the misguided and patriarchal notion that there is not enough to go around— not enough beauty, not enough male attention, and not enough success. A patriarchal worldview teaches us to view men's leadership as a given; we don't question our male colleagues' often unfettered path to the top, but we scramble over the leftover positions, as if there is only room enough at the leadership table for a few chosen women. We toughen up along the way to professional success, or through age, and we become critics and not champions of the younger women we should be mentoring.

We succeed, and we think we are exceptional, but we forget to bring other women up with us to enjoy the view.

I see through the lies that patriarchy has taught women, and I do not participate in it. As a feminist parent, it is my responsibility to ensure that my daughter does not either. Feminist parenting means keeping our guards up against the tendency of women to compete where they could collaborate to lift all of us up. Feminist moms and dads, we need to help our girls brush off and be above the mean girls whom they will encounter because that is, unfortunately, a real syndrome. In fact, go further and teach the women of tomorrow to be their sisters' keepers. When they come home with an award or a promotion, praise them for sure, but also ask them how their gains can uplift their friends. Teach them, by example, to amplify the voices of their girlfriends or, at the very least, to not stand in their way. Universal sisterhood is a difficult concept and has not always worked, but it doesn't mean we can't be strategic allies. We can pull each other up even when we don't agree on everything.

Expect as Much from Boys as We Do from Girls

We need to replace the saying "Boys will be boys" with "Boys will be expected to be as polite, as respectful, and as considerate as girls." Feminist moms and dads, we have the unenviable task of educating our daughters about sex and our sons about sex. In the Ethiopian context in particular, the word "sex" is synonymous with shame. Women in particular are made to feel shameful for having sex, let alone for desiring or pursuing it. Feminist parenting requires us to break that mould. We must teach boys and girls to name their body parts and to recognize that as uncomfortable as it makes us, children are sexual beings who will touch and explore themselves. It's our job to refrain from interfering with the curiosity that nature has given them while teaching them the appropriate where and when of self-love.

Consent is another important consideration that can't be taught too early. I learned this the hard way. From the age of three, I have taught my daughter that her private parts are her own and that no one except her immediate care takers are allowed to look or touch her there. It didn't occur to me that my son needs the same affirmations until a certain incident at his school involving the (innocent) exploration of other little boys. We focus so much on the vulnerabilities of little girls that if we are not careful, we leave our sons wide open to not only abuse but the confusion of hormones and a seemingly uncontrollable libido. Another highly important lesson we need to teach boys in particular is the myth of men's uncontrollable desire. We are raising sentient beings who must respect women and who can think beyond sex. Feminist dads, in particular, call your boys out if they linger too long looking at women's anatomy. Feminist moms, you know it is not nice to be looked at like a piece of meat. Share your feelings with your sons, for sure, but do not plead with them to respect women out of deference to you—teach them that it is the only way in which they can respect themselves. Feminist mothers do not make excuses for sons who rape.

Feminist moms, but particularly feminist dads, please, please drill consent into the very fibres of your children's sexualities as they grow up. Tell your son to stop chasing that girl if she no longer enjoys playing with him and that real men can take no for an answer. Tell your daughter that she never under any circumstances owes a man sex. Teach her to look out for herself because there will always be men who won't hear her response, but also teach her to say what she means and to not be coy and lead men on because of the dangerous idea that women need to play hard to get. Tell your little girl that it is okay to ask out the guy or the girl that she likes. Dating and romance are all good and can be good complements to the love we have for ourselves. However, our daughters as well as our sons need to know that it is good to be alone and that only really great people are worth the heartbreak they will face one day. I ask my daughter Rekka who her best friend is, and she replies "you." If I probe harder, it will be her grandmother. But she knows I will keep asking, so she replies, "myself." A conscious feminist parent aims to raise a child who won't need even her.

Teach Women of the Future to Love Being Women

Feminist dads and moms, if your ethnicity, race, or religion is an important identifier that you teach your daughter to hold dear, also include her gender. It is the category held closest to herself and is often the only visible identifier, yet usually women hold it in the least esteem. If women battled for themselves as women the way they always have on behalf of their ethnic or religious identity, patriarchy would have fallen long ago.

Own Yourself, Woman

Feminist dads, talk to your daughters about the strong women you know. Let them know that you are not okay with sexist comments; if a man ever harasses or disrespects your daughter, make sure that there is nothing in him that reminds her of you. Because unless you are the exception, you will be the standard male she will hold all future men against. Don't accept an apology on her behalf; you don't own her. Because you love her, teach her she is complete in herself.

Because I am learning both feminist parenting as I go, I often have the thought that begins "If my dad were still around." The endings vary—"I would have this and not that"; "I never would have ended up in this relationship"; or "I would never feel unloved." I know instinctively that my feminist identity should be the antidote to the primordial longing for my father—as a woman, I have been taught that my father is the protector of my existence—but it is a battle. In an effort to pull myself up, I tell myself, in the words of Toni Morrison from her book, *A Mercy*, "Own yourself, Woman." It is easier said than done, but it has been a good lesson for me concerning the meaning of feminist parenting. Feminist moms and dads, because you love your daughters and sons and because you can't protect them forever, teach them to own themselves, mind, and body. Teach them that they can live without you.

Works Cited

Morrison, Toni. *A Mercy*. Alfred A. Knopf, 2008.

Chapter 20

Mother of Two: Reflections on Love and Loss

Nikki Petersen

Sometimes motherhood isn't exactly what we expect it to be. Max's birth was both peaceful and violent. His arrival—in just one push—didn't feel like a fight, which I knew from experience that it should have; labour with my first son, Julien, had taken twelve gruelling hours, and I had to push with every muscle in my body. This time felt too easy. One push and it was over. The nurses cleaned Max up and brought him back for us to hold. He was wrapped in a small cloth blanket and wore a tiny hat. His arms were folded on his chest; it looked like he was sleeping. But he was too small and too fragile to simply be asleep, and looking down at his tiny face, which already bore a resemblance to my partner's, I felt both love and disgust—love because I had wanted him so desperately and disgust because my body had not been capable of making life this time. This wasn't how things should have been, and I finally wept for everything that had betrayed me: the world, my body, modern medicine, and even my mind for convincing me everything would be okay.

Because nothing was okay. There's no easy way to say this: I had learned several days prior that Max had a fatal heart condition and that I would have to be induced at five months, just over halfway through the pregnancy. I would be meeting him, but he would not be alive, and he would not be coming home. I knew exactly what was going to happen, but it didn't sink in until he was resting peacefully in my arms. I would be saying hello and goodbye at the exact same time. It was the most brutal introduction I'd ever had.

And just like that, it was over. We left the maternity ward the next day with a birth certificate and the newborn toiletry kit that had been set out for us. I debated whether or not to take it with me, but in the end, I did: it was all I had left of him. The days that followed were empty, confusing, lonely, bitter, desolate. I was left with a body and a mind that constantly reminded me of what I did not have. My breasts were swollen as my milk began to come in, and my stomach still looked several months pregnant. Losing control of your body is hard to accept even when you have a healthy baby, but when there is no baby, it feels particularly unfair. I was left with all the negative effects of being a mother and none of the benefits. I was left wondering what motherhood really meant in the first place.

This was all so different from my first experience of motherhood, just over two years earlier. One day, on a brief trip to New York, it occurred to me that it had been a while since my last period. This wasn't completely abnormal for me, but I decided to take a pregnancy test all the same. Its results (and the results of twelve other tests) were positive, and the following two years of my life would be the craziest, scariest, and most beautiful I had ever experienced.

I didn't worry much about miscarriage or loss with my first pregnancy—after all, by the time I learned I was expecting, I was almost already through my first trimester. I assumed that if it happened I'd be sad, but that I'd quickly get over it. Besides, losing a pregnancy was something that only happened to other women. I hadn't even planned for this baby, so whatever happened, I'd be fine.

In the end, my first pregnancy was perfectly uneventful. My son Julien was born happy and healthy, and I was swiftly introduced to the exquisite insanity of parenthood. Like most working mothers, I juggled and ran and underslept and loved and screamed and loved some more. My apartment wasn't always clean, my e-mails weren't always perfectly crafted, but things got done. This became my definition of motherhood.

As time passed and I watched my baby grow, I started to dream about having another child. At first this desire surprised me because life as a working mom was challenging enough. But I wanted my son to have a sibling, and I wanted the chance to experience babydom without the fears of a first-time parent. I now knew the joys of raising a child and believed that they outweighed the inevitable difficulties of adding a second life to my household. It didn't take long for my partner and me to decide we were ready, and this time it was anything but a surprise. I tracked my cycle, and without fail, two pink lines showed up exactly as planned.

At our first appointment, my doctor recommended telling people about the pregnancy after the first twelve weeks when the incidence of miscarriage decreases significantly, and in my social circle, this seemed to be the norm. So without giving it so much as a second thought, I planned to do the same and keep quiet until week twelve. But then I began to feel constant, relentless nausea. I had been queasy with Julien, but I hadn't imagined I would be this ill with the second child. We had little in place to accommodate me being sick, which took its toll. I could barely work or take care of Julien or do my share of household tasks. As much as I wanted to speak up and let people know why I was feeling so awful, I continued to feel an immense amount of social pressure as other women I knew waited to announce their pregnancies. I felt I could only tell a handful of close friends and family members I was expecting, so in addition to feeling sick, I felt isolated. I wondered how many women—even those who weren't confined to the couch—had experienced a similar sense of isolation in the first trimester: having to make excuses for dashing out of meetings, cancelling social engagements, or not being able to ask for a seat on the subway when they needed it. And I began to wonder why this baby wasn't allowed to exist, even though he was the size of a poppy seed, and why society expected me to be a parent of one for the first trimester, regardless of how horrible or wonderful I felt. Wouldn't it be an incredible act of feminism to open up this conversation? Perhaps, but I did not feel brave enough, as if my pregnancy weren't a "real" pregnancy yet, so instead I began to resent this baby whose existence put me in this grey area of parenting that I didn't know what to do with. But I clung to the excitement of the three-month scan: the moment when I would get to see my future child and tell the world and when, hopefully, the nausea would begin to subside.

Weeks later, my partner and I were at the hospital watching the ultrasound monitor and admiring the absurd grace of the tiny creature in my belly. It was somehow even more wonderful than it had been during my first pregnancy, as now I knew what this baby would someday become. I felt like his mother, and I wanted the world to know, which reaffirmed my belief that women should feel free to share their motherhood at any stage.

Then, the doctor broke the news that would change everything: the scan revealed a buildup of fluid behind the baby's neck.

I knew what that could mean: Down's or Patau's syndrome; some other chromosomal abnormality; or, perhaps, another problem as yet unfamiliar to me. Immediately, all the questions I'd had about how I would manage life with two young children were replaced with far graver concerns: would my child be able to say "Mama," make friends, or play sports? Would he go to college, get a job, live on his own? Would he be happy? Would I? And if he didn't survive, would it even matter, since for the world around me, he never existed in the first place?

Waiting for the results of the next round of tests, I decided to discuss our distress with our inner circle and hope for the best. I needed the support. I needed to feel like a mom, no matter what. There were so many possible outcomes. But forty-eight hours later, the doctor called to let us know that everything looked normal. She suggested a heart scan in a month or so but urged us not to worry. She also told us we were having a boy.

The next month and a half was a blur. My family came for Christmas, and we walked around Paris shopping, eating, and visiting museums. I started catching up on work, and we went away for a weekend in Normandy. Life felt exquisitely ordinary. My belly grew, and I bought myself some new maternity clothes. We began telling everyone we were expecting our second son. I felt relieved that finally this baby had a place in the world. I imagined what it would be like to raise two little boys and how I would teach them tolerance and respect and love. We picked a name: Max. Day after day, the trauma of what could have been grew more and more distant, and the prospect of becoming a mother of two became more and more real. I started to feel him move and kick. I wondered what he would look like. I pulled out my old baby books, and I hummed him songs in the bath. I wasn't sick or anxious—I was simply pregnant.

When the holidays were over, I called to schedule the recommended cardiac ultrasound. By this point, many people were excited for us, and I went to the appointment equally excited to see my baby. But this time, the doctor couldn't see the right half of his heart, and my partner and I knew by his silence that this story wasn't going to have a happy ending. We held onto our last ounce of hope until the doctor officially announced the news. There was nothing they could do, he told us. The room was quiet for a while, and we sat in stillness. I didn't believe him, didn't believe this could be happening. I searched desperately for a way to fix this, but it wasn't a fixable problem.

It was too late to perform surgery, the doctor said, so they would have to induce delivery in a matter of days. "Delivery" sounded like an exciting word, but I knew that this time, it wasn't. I was going to meet my baby, but he wasn't going to be alive. It was impossible for any of this to sink in: after all, the genetic specialist had told us everything was going to be okay.

I wondered then, as I'm sure so many women have, if there was anything I could have done to prevent this. I was told that what happened was entirely a fluke, yet I couldn't help but think otherwise. Was it my yoga class or the fever I had contracted or a chemical in my shampoo? Was something wrong with me? With my genes, with my eggs? But sadly, there was nothing to blame.

That weekend I found myself in the maternity ward. The sounds and machines and anxious fathers in the waiting room were as I had remembered from my first pregnancy. There were mothers-to-be with bellies twice the size of mine walking the halls, breathing through their contractions. A woman stared at me, and I imagined her wondering what I could possibly be doing there. To be honest, I was wondering the same thing. I felt I didn't belong. It was too soon; I wasn't ready, and it wasn't natural. I questioned the hospital's decision to put me in the maternity ward, but the midwife explained: women who lose their babies are mothers, too.

But was I? I continued to wonder. After all, I wouldn't actually be parenting this child. I would simply be saying hello and goodbye. I thought about Julien and what I told him about this baby we would never really know. Although he was only two years old, I decided it was important to talk to him about this and about what it meant. After all, he thought he was going to have a little brother. I explained to him that his brother was sick and wouldn't be able to come live with us and that he was going back to the place he came from, maybe somewhere in the sky. "Who is going to be his mama now?" Julien asked. The truth is, I didn't know.

The birth itself was difficult. We are able, as women, to muster an incredible amount of strength when giving birth. During labour with my first son, the excitement of meeting him and of bringing life into the world gave me the courage to endure absurd amounts of pain and then to smile immediately afterwards. This time, I was bringing death into the world, and my body knew it. The pain, sharp and wild, was entirely without purpose: I would never bring this baby home, or breastfeed, or wake up with him at night. He would never grow into a chubby infant or a moody toddler or an energetic, cheerful eight-year-old. All that he would be—all that he had ever been—was a fetus the size of a small cantaloupe. Perhaps he'd heard my voice sometimes; maybe he was rocked to sleep as I walked to work or swam laps at the pool, but that was all. As I moved through my contractions, I heard the cries of a newborn in the next room. I will never be able to put into words how cruel that felt.

And just like that, it was over, and I was released back into the world. There was no instruction manual on how to say goodbye, and the grief was strange and profound. I wasn't quite mourning someone I knew, yet I had carried this little person, and I'd held him in my arms. I was his mother.

I returned from the hospital to a house that seemed empty, even though it wasn't any emptier than it had been before. As I was flooded with feelings of loss, I wondered about all the women who miscarry in their first trimester, privately and without the support or acknowledgment of the wider world. As a society, we seem to consider losing a pregnancy before twelve weeks insignificant—we expect women to pick up and keep going. There is a taboo against talking about a pregnancy lost at any stage, but why? Maybe it's because there is an assumption that women will not want to talk about it or that they will feel sad or ashamed. But the feminist in me wonders why should we be ashamed and why shouldn't we be allowed to grieve? When a friend or family member dies, we don't keep it to ourselves—the world acknowledges our grief. Perhaps, there isn't as much to remember when a pregnancy is lost, but there's a lot to say goodbye to. Of course, it is possible to try for another child, redirecting hopes and dreams toward a new little person, but this will never replace a prior loss—nor should we want it to.

I began to think about all the people who had known I was pregnant: my family and friends, of course, but also my colleagues, clients, and employees; the teachers at my son's daycare; my pharmacist; and even the barista at my regular coffee shop. I had thought I was in the safe zone, well into my second trimester, and had never imagined having to share this kind of news. In my sadness, fear, and shame, it was an overwhelming task to tell them all. But I began. Some I told directly. Others were told by mutual friends and acquaintances. Then I posted something on Facebook.

In a matter of days, my inbox was full of messages from hundreds of women telling me that they, too, had lost a pregnancy—some as early as six weeks, others as late as forty. Their stories were different, but they all had one thing in common: these women still thought about the babies they never got a chance to know. Not necessarily often and not necessarily in a life-altering way, but all of these unborn children had a place in their mothers' minds. As I read message after message from friends and family, I was stunned by how many of these stories were new to me. Close friends had miscarried and never told anyone but their partner. Some just didn't know how to talk about it, they said. Some didn't feel legitimate in their sadness and wondered at what point do we consider a baby a baby? Others kept the experience to themselves out of a desire for privacy or a sense of embarrassment, or in the hope that they could simply forget and move on. I can relate to all of those feelings: if we had lost our son before twelve weeks, I'm sure only a handful of people would have known.

In retrospect, I'm glad people knew because working through the grief without the outpouring of love I received would have been unthinkable. Flowers and gifts and cards arrived from all over the world. People came over to help us cook and clean and watch Julien so my partner and I could take time to mourn. I received heartfelt letters from the doctors who had treated me throughout the pregnancy. I cried with the daycare teachers and the barista. It sometimes felt strange or uncomfortable or surreal, but my little world, in its way, was grieving with me. It wasn't all easy: some good friends didn't reach out—I assume because they didn't know what to say—and that stung. But overall, I felt a profound sense of support.

I wish I could say that this fixed everything, but the months following the birth and death of our son were more difficult than I ever could have anticipated. It felt like the world had cheated me. I had to lose the baby weight, but every session at the gym was a reminder of the injustice of the world. I had to return to work, yet the state of my hormones left me emotional and anxious, unable to concentrate or find joy in my job. Both my mind and body kept me from moving on as swiftly as I had hoped.

Today, although I don't consider myself recovered—or even know what that would mean—I'm beginning to accept the reality of the situation: this happened, it's awful, and, no, it isn't fair.

There isn't any way to find a reason for what happened; there is no neat conclusion to this story. I don't believe that Max was brought into the world to teach me something. But I do believe we can grow from situations like these, and I've gained a new perspective on what it means to be a mother and the way we as a society conceive of pregnancy and react to its loss. I believe we deserve to tell our stories unapologetically, and I believe opening up the discussion on miscarriage and stillbirth is a magnificent act of feminism. This is precisely why I decided to share my story. I would like to encourage other women to take a leap of faith and talk about their experiences with loss. One day, I hope we'll live in a world where women feel free to share the progress of their pregnancies, come what may, a world where feminism means accepting the realities so many women face. At the end of the day, all women who carry children are mothers if they so desire and deserve to be treated as such, regardless of the outcome. Maybe, motherhood starts when we want it to. On the hard days, I remind myself of this: I am still the mother of two kids, just not in the way I expected.

Chapter 21

From Dreams to Action: Creating My Own Happily Ever After by Choosing to Adopt as a Young, Single Woman

Astrid Rosemary Ndagano Haas

> "Teach her about difference. Make difference ordinary. Make difference normal."
> —Adichie 59

The Decision: Defining My Dream

I decided the time was right for me to become a mom when I was twenty-nine, except I was not going to become a mom the conventional way. I was single and had been for most of my life. I was doing well in my career. I travelled the world quite a bit; in fact, that was one of my favourite things to do. Perhaps, however, most unconventional of all, given where I was in life, was that I decided I was going to adopt.

My dream has always been to adopt. However, I thought that I would be going through the process later in life, as many people who make this decision do. It was going to be at the point where I had a husband, a house, and a dog. In essence, I was planning to go the route of adoption in what perhaps seemed the more traditional way. Why was this? Well, as much as I had a desire to adopt, I will be the first to admit that I was strongly conditioned by so-called chick flicks. In those films—I started watching Disney princesses and then moved on to romantic comedies (rom-coms)—a single, usually quite desperate woman, whose life is chaotic, meets the man of her dreams and all the pieces fall into place. Then, even if the relationship does not work out right from the start, they find a way, and, in the end, they live happily ever after. In my mind, I extended the scene further, as I always knew that a big part of my happily ever after would be the bit beyond the film where they have children. So I waited and waited, sometimes impatiently, for my own Prince Charming to ride to me through the sunset and for my own happily ever after to begin.

But it didn't—at least not like I thought it was supposed to. In fact, it was far from what was in the films. I had a wonderful group of friends, a very supportive and loving family, and a great education and, as noted, I was travelling the world. In most respects, I had what from the outside was a wonderful and privileged life. Yet I was only able to dwell on one thing: my constant singleness. As I got older, it got so bad that it manifested itself in the form of clinical depression—I have no qualms in admitting this. I hated myself because I could not work out what was wrong with me, why no one could love me. I spent long days and nights trying to figure out how I could change myself so that someone would finally be able to love me. It did not help that I was emotionally bullied when I was a teenager in school, being often called "a loser." The more it did not happen, the worse it got, and, finally, the only logical conclusion I could come to was that those bullies in high school were right: I was indeed a loser.

In the meantime, friends around me were having their own happily ever after, and I gallivanted around the world to their beautiful weddings. I was genuinely very happy for them. But with each wedding, I was wondering when it would finally be my turn. People kept saying to me, "Don't worry. I am sure it will happen for you" or "It will happen when you least expect it." The problem was that I could not "least expect it" anymore; it was front and centre to my life, and I became convinced that all I needed to find eternal happiness was a man.

After many of years of suffering and my condition worsening, I decided it was time to get help. I am a perfectionist, and it takes a lot for me to ask for help. Particularly in this case because I truly believed that there was nothing clinically wrong with me; no one could help someone not be a loser. Finally, and thankfully, through cajoling from some lovely friends and family who cared deeply for me, I found a wonderful psychologist who helped me think and see outside the proverbial hole I had dug myself. I also started reading again, which is one of my favourite pastimes but something I had not kept up with during the height of my depression. Reading was very important, as it helped me gain some perspective outside the rom-coms I tortured myself with when I was depressed.

After years of working on myself, I was finally able to once again clear the fog and engage in self-reflection. I realized that there was no one else responsible for my happiness but myself. Although this may sound very simple, it was perhaps one of the most difficult realizations I had to come to in life. This was also the time I decided that I was a feminist because I did not need to conform to societal norms of women to find my happiness. I was not only a feminist but a proud feminist, who had to take care of myself and my own internal happiness. The realization that trying to achieve conformity had harmed me was deeply shocking. Being able to finally embrace my feminist identity supported me in other parts of my life too, particularly in my career. Once I had managed this step, I was finally able to pursue my own happily ever after. I decided to try and dissect what my dreams and aspirations were so that I could start putting them into action.

From this, I realized that although I had dwelled on the fact that my happily ever after was marriage, my dream was actually to have children. Thinking through this, I realized that I had always associated having children with finding the perfect man, building the perfect house, and having the perfect life. I finally recognized that I did not actually know what "perfect" meant in this sense; rather, I had to discover what perfect was for myself. Therefore, I went ahead and put my own dreams into action and became a mom.

The Journey: Realizing My Dream

When I decided to go down the path of adoption, I had braced myself for many things: immense bureaucracy, long waits, as well as the toughness of being a single parent. The one thing I did not expect, which was possibly the toughest part of the whole process, was how openly judgmental people were about my decision to adopt as a young, single mother. Today, as I sit here and write this piece with my most special, wonderful baby daughter napping in the background, I am forever grateful that I did not listen to them. Rather, I am deeply fulfilled with the journey of adoption because it has made me a much stronger woman and better feminist parent to my daughter.

In order to understand my journey, it is important to illuminate some of the judgments I have experienced. In hindsight, it would have been very helpful to know more about the ways that society thinks about a single woman adopting a child and to have been able to prepare myself for what was coming my way rather than, perhaps ignorantly, assuming that everyone would be happy with my decision. None of the parenting books or adoption books I read mentioned this challenge. To support other women who may make a similar decision in the future, I share a set of responses I perhaps should have given at the time:

> Comment: Have you really thought it through? Are you sure you are old enough to make that decision? Why don't you wait a few years until the perfect man comes along?

> What my response should have been: Actually, now that you mention it, after having been old enough to vote for more than ten years; after having lived, studied, and worked in eight different countries on three continents; after having been financially stable and independent since university; after having decided to go perhaps the most difficult route to have a child, with my life and future parenting skills being mercilessly critiqued by the government and social workers; and after having to wait more than two years, to have my child—maybe you are right, and I have not thought my decision through.

Not only did I put pressure on myself to conform to the idea that I needed to marry before having children, society also pressured me to conform as well. Society expects women to have children, yet society, at the same time, restricts how it can be done. Aside from not understanding why I chose to become a mother as a single woman, people found my decision to adopt even more controversial. I was told a number of times that even in-vitro fertilization from a sperm donor was more acceptable than adoption.

Comment: Now you are just advertising your infertility.

What my response should have been: Really? That is news to me.

This comment was perhaps one of the most culturally centred comments I received. In Uganda, producing children is a sign of a woman's status. In fact, the verb "to produce" is actually used when it comes to children. When a woman has twins, for example, her worth, in terms of her dowry, increases as she is perceived to be more fertile. In Uganda, we have some of the highest fertility rates in the world. However, due to high costs of raising children, a large number of children in Uganda are placed in orphanages to receive care; others are abandoned.

Even with this mandate and expectation of women having many children in Uganda, adoption is still seen as a last resort for those women are ostensibly unable to produce. That I was choosing adoption at a young age was seen by people as giving up on having children of my own. I do not know whether I will have biological children or not. In the future, if the right partner comes along, then I may, only if to experience the feeling of pregnancy and birth. But I may also just choose to adopt again.

Comment: You know, now you will never get married.

What my response should have been: Oh thank goodness.

When I mentioned my astonishment about how many people have criticized my decision to adopt, I am told, "I am sure that's just a cultural thing." It was not. Such comments came from all kinds of people from different backgrounds, men and women alike. Given my background, it is perhaps the one that, at first, pushed my sensitive buttons the most.

However, I believe that these comments and experiences have better prepared me if I should choose to partner someday. If a man does not respect me as a single mother by adoption, then I know they are not the right person for me. It took this journey of self-realization and becoming a parent to understand that protecting my daughter's and my own preciousness is worth more than any partner in the world to me. As much as I may still want to marry and for my daughter to have a father, if a prospective partner does enter our lives, but he does not bring joy to our lives, then he is not worth it and we will do just fine by ourselves.

Comment: But your career is going so well, why don't you wait for a bit. This may not be good for it.

What my response should have been: Oh does that mean you think that my career is going to go less well in the future?

I am sure that this is a comment that not only single mothers get but all women who are considering having children in general. Long before I pursued my path of parenthood, I received an important piece of advice from a woman I respect greatly. She is quite a bit older than me and ended up not having children, not because she did not want to but because she was always waiting for the perfect time. She decided to wait for that elusive optimal time to come along, putting her career first. In the end, she woke up one day and found that she was too old to fulfil her dream of having children. She advised me, therefore, that there is no ideal time in your life; instead, you make it ideal by resetting your priorities and working around it.

At the time I started my adoption process, my career was indeed going well. I had finally found my passion workwise. In the two years that I waited for my daughter's arrival, my career only got better. On top of it all, unlike pregnancy, where you have approximately nine months' notice for your baby's arrival, with adoption you are unsure when the call will come that will change your life forever. For me, the call came after I had just come back from a two-week trip to Myanmar and the U.S. and I was home for a break before I would be travelling again in the following weeks.

Before my baby came along, I worked insane hours as I only had to focus on myself and my career. However, I realized that it was not wholly fulfilling to me. I have only been a mother for a short while at the time of writing this, so there is still a lot for me to discover. I will say that I was absolutely terrified of being a parent, being a single parent, and of being solely responsible for a little life. Many people told me that I was in for a difficult ride as a single parent. Some made it seem that it would be near impossible. When my daughter entered my life, I braced myself for beautiful but difficult times. However, what I have discovered is that mothering comes naturally to me. My instincts are there to help and to guide me. And with family and friends surrounding me, I am never doing it alone. I know that things will change, particularly when I return to work, and I realize motherhood will mean letting go of some of my commitments. Nonetheless, I feel my life has become so much more fulfilling. Becoming a mother has made me a more rounded person. I also believe that if my career was going well before my daughter, there should be no reason why it should not continue this way, particularly because I am a far happier person than I was before. I fully recognize the challenges I will face as a single and employed mother. However, I now know I have the strength to face these challenges.

The Future: Our Long Path Ahead, Together

My path has not only gifted me with an amazing daughter, it has also made me a strong feminist parent. With this, I am confident I am now able to give my daughter a more robust foundation in life based on the lessons I have learned; this includes how to have a healthy sense of self as well as how to openly and assertively reject insensitive and judgmental remarks. Moving forwards, I want to live our life together drawing upon suggestions from the feminist manifesto I live by—namely *Dear Ijeawele, or A Feminist Manifesto in Fifteen Suggestions* by Chimamanda Ngozi Adichie. The final section of this paper, therefore, is a set of solemn promises to my daughter on how we will pursue this together.

> 1. "Teach her (that) the idea of 'gender roles' is absolute nonsense." (Adichie 15)

Red was always my favourite colour. I also like bright yellow, orange, blue, and green. Although I will also sometimes wear pink, it is not something I am immediately drawn to. Therefore, less to break gender stereotypes and more to dress my daughter in colours I like, I went out to find her clothes in those colours. I was genuinely astounded that in 2018, this is still a difficult undertaking. Most of the shops are organized in two sections: one in blue for the boys and the other in pink for the girls. To challenge gendered clothing, I bought my daughter clothes from both sections. This was my first and hard lesson on how to overcome these predefined norms.

Most challenges still await me, as my daughter is still only a few months old; she is more interested in staring at my multicoloured bedcovers than any particular piece of clothing. However, I have already begun to prepare for the future. For example, I have ensured that my daughter will have a wide array of toys and books, particularly ones about notable women— Favilli and Cavallo's *Good Night Stories for Rebel Girls* being my current favourite. I believe that in our home life, together, we will be able to achieve this. The major question for me is how this will develop once she enters playgroups, kindergarten, and school. It is not that I don't want my daughter to be a so-called girly girl. I just want her to be able to choose that rather than have society choose for her.

2. "Beware of the danger of what I call Feminism Lite.... Being a feminist is like being pregnant. You either are or you are not. You either believe in full equality of men and women or you do not." (Adichie 20)

Being a mom is pretty much equivalent to being a teacher. It is also means becoming a student again. Each child, even as an infant, is different. Everyone's situation is different. Therefore, I continue to learn from my daughter every day about her needs and my own, too. One thing that becoming a mother has taught me is that being a feminist is not a label one can just carry sometimes. It is true that women are progressing in the world, but we are still far from reaching anything close to gender parity. The reason why, in the past, I did not want to be labelled a feminist was because the term carried some negative connotations. I used to believe there were much more important things to strive for in the world. However, now I know that if I am not a true feminist and do not aspire to full feminist values, then none of the other dreams and aspirations I have for my daughter will happen. Therefore, by being a proud feminist parent, I want to build these foundations for her. One of the major lessons I want to pass on to her is that there is no such thing as feminism lite; rather, I want her, unlike me, to grow up and fight for her rights and equality right from the start.

3. "Never speak of marriage as an achievement." (Adichie 30)

A major mistake I have made in my life that I want my daughter to avoid is to assume that happiness can only be found in marriage. She has taught me that you can pursue your dreams as an individual and find happiness through self-love and care. Even today, I am told the more determined and independent I become, the less likely it will be I will ever get married. However, if I had not become the strong, independent feminist I am today, then I might never have pursued my dreams and ambitions and I would not be with my daughter. I would have also likely failed at finding happiness because right now, since becoming a mom, I have felt the happiest and the most content I have ever been. Therefore, my success in parenting will be evident if I can raise a daughter who has the ability to think for herself and who does not worry about what others think. If I am able to do this, then I am sure she will not see marriage as women's only potential achievement but rather as merely another option for her if she wishes.

> 4. "Teach her to reject likeability. Her job is not to make herself likeable, her job is to be her full self, a self that is honest and aware of the equal humanity of other people." (Adichie 36)

Until reading *Dear Ijeawele*, I had never really reflected on this part of my self. It was one of those illuminating moments that provided deep insight into myself. I have tried to make myself likeable. I would back down from something I truly believed in if I felt that it would make me less popular. I felt I failed if someone decided they did not like me or a decision I took. This quality, I now see, is one that we consciously or subconsciously pass on to most girls, no matter the negative affect on their self-esteem.

I am just learning for myself that likeability is not an achievement in itself. If there is something I truly believe, I realize that I must pursue it, even if someone does not like me for doing so. Although it took me a long time to get here, I know that in raising my daughter, I will not require her to be likeable just to please others.

Dreams for My Daughter

Drawing upon inspiration from Adichie, I decided that I wanted to immortalize my own promises to my daughter in a letter. Therefore, between receiving the phone call that she had arrived and the day she came home, I wrote her a letter to honour the fact that she made my dreams come true and to enshrine my dreams for her. This is part of the letter I wrote:

> To the most special daughter in the world,
>
> After nearly two years of working to put my dreams of becoming a Mama into action, the time has finally come for you to come

Activist Engagements with Pacifist Roots

My family is the classic Western European one. I am a white heterosexual mother of three girls (fourteen, sixteen, and nineteen years old at the time of writing this paper), and I live with my partner, the father of the children. Writing this chapter has made me revisit the path of parenting my partner and I chose, built, and improvised together.

The combination of feminism and ecology is a transversal theme on this path. When looking for its roots, I recognize the importance of my origins. I grew up in the countryside in a Protestant family in Germany during the Cold War. In the south of Germany, where I lived, American troops were stationed. In the Western German imagination, we were at the centre of the international arms race. A Third World War was perceived as a real threat, as we believed that Western Europe was lodged between the two main actors of the Cold War—U.S. and the U.S.S.R.— with most of their weapons' targets converging in this area. The pacifist movement was, therefore, strong and had ramifications at the local level, also on the country-side. As military service was still obligatory for young men, the question was necessarily an issue for us as teenagers: young men had to decide if they did their military service (which meant for us, preparing for war) or if they wanted to opt for a civil service, after undergoing an exam as "conscientious objectors." In this context, the pacifist movement engaged in not only the deconstruction of hegemonic structures from an international level (the U.S. dominating NATO, but also U.S. and the U.S.S.R. fighting for influence in the Third World) down to the meso- and micro-level but also in the construction of new, alternative models of a pacifist society, with feminism and ecology among its pillars. I was involved in this movement as a teenager, and this activism forged my personal and political values. One of the first big protest marches I participated in was against the deployment of American Pershing missiles on German soil, and I walked with my friends under the banner of feminism, as feminists were among the key stakeholders of the pacifist movement.

When I began thinking about parenthood, I was already in my thirties. I was working as a freelance consultant and had started some teaching assignments at a university. My partner and I were then living in a small village in the French countryside, where a considerable network of people tried to live a healthy rural life at the margins of the liberal economy through reducing water and energy consumption as well as buying locally grown organic food. We were engaged in the growing antiglobalization movement where I found a similar convergence of different causes.

The Choice of the Way to Give Birth as the Entry into Feminist Parenting

The choice of a natural birth was important to me, as it cohered with our lifestyle. For our first child, the midwife considered a birth at our home too risky, since the local maternity service had closed a couple of months before and the next closest one was at least forty-five minutes of windy road away. We, therefore, went to a "birth house" (*maison de naissance*[2]) with a midwife present and no medicalized features (which is exceptional in France where giving birth is generally medicalized); hospital facilities, though, were only five minutes away, just in case. My partner was present all the time while the midwife explained everything; he felt very much involved. We had a room with a double bed, and when the baby was born, all three of us could snuggle together.

The two other girls were born at home. The third birth took place in autumn; the midwife had an hour to drive, under bad weather conditions. The birth was exceptionally fast, compared to the first two, and as a result, the midwife was still on the road when the baby arrived. A colleague of the midwife gave instructions by phone; my partner who had vivid memories of the two former births actively assisted. This was obviously an intense moment for the three of us.

Reflecting on feminist parenting, I believe the way these births took place was crucial. As giving birth at home is rare in France, our choice was strongly questioned, and we had to justify ourselves. The births had a clear link with ecology, as they took place in a natural way. Besides ecology, the other reason for the homebirths was self-determination: the idea (forged by many testimonies I had read and heard[3]) of being commanded by medical staff while giving birth in a maternity ward was horrifying to me. And I wanted the father to be engaged in the process of giving birth. My partner played an active role in every birth, even a crucial one for the third birth. He now considers that these births acted as a decisive entry for him into parenthood; he became a significant actor right from the start. Through these births, I felt that I was able to live my feminism.

Moreover, I did not want a medicalized birth. Through years of practicing yoga, I had developed a fairly good knowledge of my body, which helped me to tackle pain. My decision also had a lot to do with my desire to stay in control during birth rather than being under the control of others.

From Sexual Partners to Joined Parenthood

I had been with my partner for four years before our first child was born. During this period and after the births, he accepted voluntarily my wish not to take the pill, which I rejected for ecological reasons but also because I never had succeeded in taking it regularly, making it inefficient. Every morning, I took my temperature to calculate my fertile days, during which we used condoms to prevent pregnancy. It helped me to know my body and made us share responsibilities in a way that was convenient for us. Looking back now, this shared responsibility concerning contraception seems to have prepared the ground for shared parenthood. We spoke about it recently and to my great surprise, my partner could not at all remember the thermometer next to the bed, the paper and the pencil to record daily findings, or my calculations to decide whether or not we needed a condom.[4] As he tends to have quite a selective memory, I interpret this forgetfulness as a sign that this was not a problem for him, probably also because I did all the measuring and calculating.

My partner's presence during the natural births of our daughters has changed the perspective he had of my body. During the first birth (which was very long and tedious), the young midwife was responding to my partner's many questions. He followed closely the appearance of the baby's head in the vagina, the way the midwife liberated her neck from the umbilical cord with a flick of the wrist, and even some unpleasant side effects, such as some feces appearing during the last part of the baby's expulsion (which is avoided in hospitals through enemas). As my perineum was torn a bit, the midwife put in some stitches and explained the technique for capturing the different layers of tissue to my partner, who watched attentively. He was obviously in a special state, as he usually avoids looking at any bleeding wound. For the second birth, my state was not new to him, and he could get more involved around the baby; he put the knot into the umbilical cord, which shaped forever our second daughter's belly button. During the third birth, we were alone at the moment the baby arrived, which was not planned. He played an active role and had to replace the midwife. For example, he had to check if the umbilical cord was around her neck before the expulsion, and a little later he had to oversee the expulsion of the placenta. This obviously gave him a look at my body that was completely disconnected from sexuality, seduction, and arousal. During this whole time, he was in a special state, high on adrenaline, I suppose. He actually cried when the baby was delivered and when her colour got a bit more pinkish and other signs showed that she was fine. He was exalted when the midwife finally arrived and confirmed that all was well.

Through these births our sexuality has changed not only because of physical changes that induce different sensations but also because of the different perspectives he has now of my body. I have the impression that sexuality has changed also because we are able to speak more openly about our bodies and their functions after these births. More generally, these three births were intense shared experiences, which strongly brought us together. Our sexuality became more mature as a result and, all in all, better.

Mobile, Ecological Babies

The early childhood years of our girls were another crucial phase in which we had to take many decisions, which were often influenced by our surroundings. For example, I breastfed each child for about a year and a half, which, most of all, was a practical issue for me. I could be mobile with the baby and take her anywhere. I could be flexible about the time and place of the feeding, and not be overregulated by the feeding schedule of the infant. This worked because I breastfed anywhere, which was quite usual in a German setting, but it triggered some surprising reactions in France. While teaching, I managed to express milk to store for future longer absences, which required quite a bit of logistics considering hygiene, as expressing milk in a place like a university toilet was not always easy. I also took two of my girls to Madagascar where I went quite often for short term professional missions at this period. They were about one year old, and each time childcare had been organized locally. Deciding to take them with me was obviously not just linked to breastfeeding; it was more generally a good compromise for me, as I do not think that I would have left them alone at their age for three or four weeks. I perceived breastfeeding and these kind of arrangements as giving me some freedom as a mother, allowing me to go back to work gradually and quite early.

There was obviously also an ecological component to the choice of breastfeeding: we tried hard to bring our girls up as much as possible protected from chemicals and other potentially harmful substances, and breastfeeding seemed the best solution to this during the first months of their lives.

Ecological concern was also the main reason that we used cloth diapers (at least when we were home); they did need washing and drying, but they produced so much less waste than conventional diapers. We actually ordered them in Germany, as they were hard to find in France at the time. When we were moving about for more than a couple of hours, we tried to use unbleached conventional diapers, as bleaching is a toxic process and quite useless from our point of view (Why should diapers be shining white?). At the time, there was only one German brand selling these diapers, and they were terribly expensive in France and hard to find. We, therefore, took dozens of packages of diapers with us every time we came back from Germany; the car was often filled up to the rim with the bulky packs.

For me, these were my choices (and, as far as I can tell, were not the result of outside pressure), and they were compromises that allowed us to keep a certain control over how and what the babies were exposed to and consumed. Feminist literature and also some feminist friends are quite critical about this way of living motherhood. Breastfeeding has been stigmatized as a form of submission to masculine domination, among others by Elisabeth Badinter, who is a well-known French feminist. She considers that breastfeeding means putting the babies' needs before the mothers'. Rather than as a submission to the norms of socially sanctioned motherhood, I experienced this period as a personal affirmation of my choice to mother at the crossroads of ecology and feminism.

A Stay-at-Home Father

Another critical issue in my feminist parenting concerned my partner stopping employed work after the birth of our second daughter, whereas I continued working fulltime (partly working from home). This choice was not guided by an apprehension about childcare, as we did consider that it was good for our children to socialize with others; and good-quality childcare facilities were available. For children under three years of age, we were entitled to receive subsidies for paying a nanny, and all-day public facilities were available for free from three years old. It was rather a choice based on our life project, especially considering housing. My partner used this time at home not mainly on childcare, but mostly on "building a comfortable nest". After we bought a small old house, he started building by himself a large extension, using untreated wood and other ecological materials. He also engaged in the parents' association at the local school and became an elected member of the local community council. He was invested in the girls' childhood more than most fathers, as it was often him that brought the children to school or fetched them in the early evening.

The house extension advanced slowly, and as the girls grew older, my partner experienced the classical "housewife syndrome": since he did not have a formal paying job, in many people's minds, he did nothing. Having a father with no recognised social role was sometimes an issue for our children, who had to explain that "he does not work", even though they saw him engaged in many activities. Being a perfectionist in his workmanship, he spent over a dozen years on building the extension. As the years went by, he suffered more and more from the lack of recognition from society (including from the neighbours and the extended family); he became frustrated and sometimes depressed. He was also more and more interested in gender; he read more about it and asked many questions. With one of his friends (who was deeply affected by a recent breakup), he started a men's group, who meets twice a month to discuss issues of masculinity.

Now that the girls have started to "leave the nest," he finds this transition difficult. He wants to go back to a working life now, not only because the girls need more financial support during their studies but also because he is experiencing the empty nest syndrome.

whereas in Germany, where working mothers of small children used to be called disapprovingly "raven mothers," I could hold up the largely free public childcare facilities (at lot more available in France than in Germany) as giving me the option to continue to work. And in a way, it was the combination of aspirations forged in my youth in Germany and the possibilities offered in the French welfare state that made my choices possible. Ecology has been an important yet difficult principle, even more so for my partner than myself, to strike a balance with feminism; it has not always been easy and is still a constant subject of discussion between me, my partner, and our daughters. In this complex context, self-determination has clearly been the key to my feminist parenting based on the humanist values of solidarity, equality, tolerance, and ecology.

For those who wonder about their entry point into feminist parenting, I suggest you find out what you really want and then build towards it with your partner through open communication. Also, talk to parents whose parenting seems inspiring, read books, question your own parents, look for midwifes with whom you connect, but do what you feel confident doing, down in your guts. Team up with your partner right from the start and share as much as possible—chores, emotions, ideas—in line with your political opinions and your worldview. I am convinced that feminist parenting will potentially have a profound political impact on our common future.

Endnotes

1. An interesting overview of this tendency has been published by Mediapart (Feb. 12 2018): "Entre alterféminisme et antiféminisme, la droite tâtonne."
2. Only a few of these "birth houses" existed in France and were managed by associations of parents. They became illegal around 2000.
3. At the time, I had never been hospitalized, and I must admit that the idea of going into hospital made me afraid. This is important to underline, as many people thought it courageous to give birth at home.
4. I admire today's mobile phone apps that do most of these calculations for women (like Fertility Friend Ovulation, which is interestingly

advertised as a means to help you getting pregnant, not as a way to know when you need contraception). I learned of their existence from my girls, who are using them.

Works Cited

Badinter, Elisabeth. *Le conflit, la femme et la mère.* Flammarion, 2010.

Delaporte, Lucie. *Entre alterféminisme et antiféminisme, la droite tâtonne.* Mediapart, February 12, 2018, www.mediapart.fr/journal/france/120218/entre-alterfeminisme-et-antifeminisme-la-droite-tatonne?onglet=full. Accessed 22 Feb. 2020.

Chapter 23

Why I Have Decided Not to Parent (and Why I Won't Regret It)

Elizabeth Wright Veintimilla

Gaining Control in a Patriarchal World

The decision not to parent holds a great amount of power and privilege. The vast majority of women worldwide—especially those who experience multiple layers of identity-based oppression—don't have control over their own sexual and reproductive health. I do, which is why I can write this chapter in the first place. Feminism to me has become a lens through which I not only view the world but also view and reflect upon my own life story, from my dreams coming true to my experiences with trauma and machismo. I see this chapter as an opportunity for me to explore and share my reasons not to have children, not as a way to justify myself to you but as a means of catharsis and relief for me.

"Well, I would ask you to reconsider, you know?" a man once said to me while talking about a (hypothetical) unplanned pregnancy and abortion. Patriarchy is a system that allows men to dominate those of us who identify as women. It makes men believe that their opinion about our body matters. It doesn't. Just because a man may have been inside my body during sex doesn't mean he should have a say over what I should do with my body. Patriarchy enforces the concept that giving birth and raising children is a woman's natural destiny and that becoming a mother is the ultimate goal in life because it will complete and fulfill women. Imposing this idea on us is one of the most violent and manipulative forms of oppression, which is why it is so hard to challenge and resist it. It has taken me a long time to recognize this and to allow myself to know that what I want in life is valid, with or without children.

Under patriarchy, women are often assigned the emotional work of caring for others, which can make it hard to prioritize ourselves. We constantly are expected to pay more attention to the feelings and needs of others and to put our own wellbeing aside, which applies not only to the private sphere, where we are expected to do all the domestic work, but also to our professional careers. It's no coincidence that most nurses, nannies, and domestic workers are women. Men who do this type of work are often stigmatized by patriarchy as well because roles that involve caring for others are gendered as feminine. The reason I address this issue here is to contextualize women's lack of agency to care for ourselves and to live autonomous lives. I have been privileged with opportunities to live on my own, and I've enjoyed it so much that I don't want to live differently. I consider myself a caring person. I care about the world and about people both within and outside of my communities. However, when it comes to my daily routine and how I use my personal time and space, I want it to be by and for myself. I am worried not only about how much of my time would go to parenting a child but also about the expenses required to parent. I do not see myself making these sacrifices ever.

From a feminist perspective, I know that motherhood does not have to be a life-stealing experience. I can be a mother and work, travel, and be an activist at the same time, partly because of my class and race privilege. I know that. There are so many mothers in my life who are so fierce with everything they do, from owning their own business and taking care of their own family (and other families) to becoming some of the most well-known feminist activists. I know how much mothers are capable of doing, mainly because I have my own mom as an example. I don't want children because I know that decision is permanent.

Kids are not even the problem to begin with. Karina Vergara Sánchez, a feminist teacher and journalist from Mexico, reflects on the argument that *les niñes* (children) steal their mothers' lives and the idea that women who mother don't have any agency. Sánchez argues that capitalism—not motherhood—steals the life and happiness of mothers because it condemns them to take care of their children and their husband, isolated from other women and in servitude (http://www.la-critica.org/opinion-las-comadres/. I agree with Sánchez's take and share her wish that those who choose motherhood can experience it with joy and in community with other women. Capitalism steals the lives of women before and regardless of motherhood. It has made me feel like I am not a priority, and that profit is more important than my own life. Capitalism also creates unhealthy and unrealistic standards of productivity and success, often making people—myself included—feel that we are not good enough or producing enough. For women, this system of power also dictates what we should and are allowed to accomplish with our lives.

All the Feels (and Fears)

I've experienced paranoia, dissociation, depression, and social anxiety at various moments of my life. I have never been diagnosed with a chronic mental illness, but my relatively short experiences with them have made it clear to me how uneasy I feel about everything, all the time. Trauma that I've experienced or witnessed has led me to feel endless fear about what could happen to my loved ones. If I know someone is on their way home and they don't text me to confirm they've arrived safely, for example, my mind will convince me that they have gotten into a car accident on the highway. I'm terrified of all the things that could happen to a potential child of mine. It's inevitable that harmful things will happen, and that's what terrifies me the most.

I've witnessed death closely enough to fear it tremendously. I fear the possibility of having a child and losing my partner, making me a widow and a single parent; I fear the possibility that if something were to happen to me, my child would become an orphan. I'm scared of something happening to my child and losing them. I picture all kinds of scenarios because they're real. Two days after my eleventh birthday, my father died of a sudden heart attack. He left for a jog and never returned. From health issues, to mass shootings, accidents, and suicide, I've witnessed a lot of death in my family and in my larger community as well. Dealing with a loved one's death is extremely painful, and I wouldn't want my own child to experience it the way I have had to. Likewise, I'm scared my child's fate is defined by genes. What can my child inherit from my family, my ancestors, and me? It could be mental patriarchy treats women not as self-sufficient people but as fragile ones.

At the same time, I don't see myself living completely alone when I'm older. I think that community, including family, can take different forms and mean different things. Community can be a particular place, a partner or a close friend. If I want to have communities and people around when I'm older, I have to build and rebuild them as time passes. I see myself being surrounded by people I've met along the way from all aspects of my life, including high school, college, work, feminist collectives, and more. Communication is becoming more and more accessible, so I'm not afraid of losing touch with those who matter. I also hope to live in the company of my current partner. Forming a family doesn't necessarily mean getting married and having children. There are different ways of doing that.

Conclusion

Reflecting on my decision not to parent in silence and solitude is one thing, but writing about it and sharing it with the world is another. I wrote this chapter with the purpose of finding relief and liberation, instead of wanting to prove myself to my readers. This process has given me a lot of strength and motivation to continue building my life the way I want and need. I am creating my path and identity outside of motherhood, and have found many ways to do that with joy, hard work, self-care, and community.

Motherhood and the mothering instinct are social constructs. I've shared my decision to never have children with other people, and their reactions are usually the same: "But what if you regret it later?" or "Well, you'd be a great mom!" My decision to not become a parent just shows that I'm building my life as carefully as possible and according to what I know is best for me and my future. "I don't want to" is a valid enough reason to not have children. I am not selfish, wrong, or alone. Parenting is a major life decision that should not be imposed on anyone by a partner, family, or the world we live in.

And no, I won't regret it.

Works cited

http://www.la-critica.org/opinion-las-comadres/

Part III

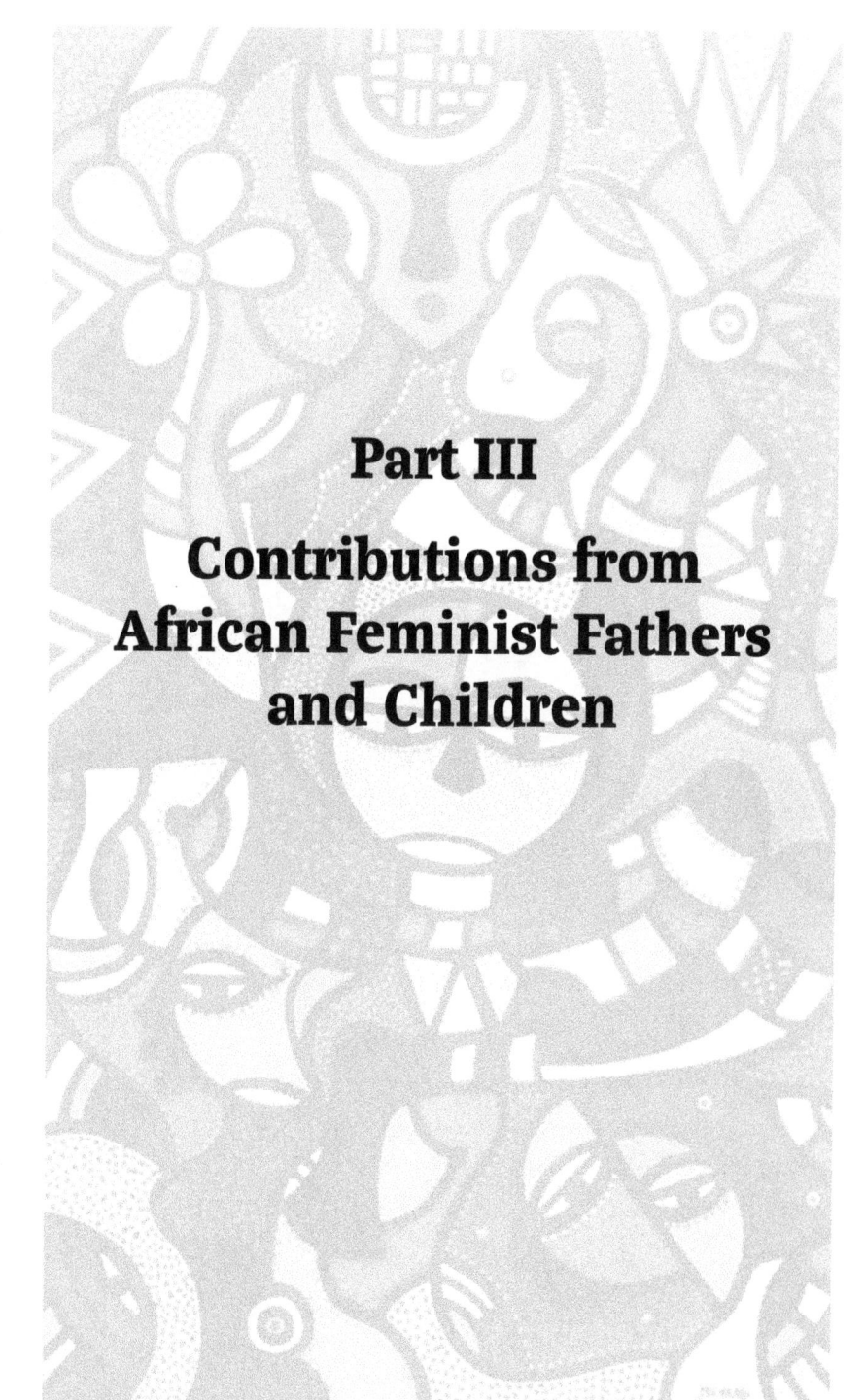

Contributions from African Feminist Fathers and Children

Chapter 24

What My Mom and My Daughter Taught Me

Cheikh "Keyti" Séne

As a forty-five-year-old Senegalese man who is the father of a ten-year-old girl, I still hesitate to call myself a feminist—not because there may be some sort of negative undertone to naming myself one or to be named as such but because it implies a way of understanding and interacting with the world that I'm not always sure I represent. I may hesitate to call myself a feminist because I don't know what it is to experience the world as a woman but I am convinced that I do not want to support any social or political system of injustice and inequality, especially when they are based on gender. Patriarchy, to name it, is a social construct that deeply affects all of society, but women and children primarily; it relies on its victims—through political, cultural, or religious practices—to perpetuate itself. However, some do escape patriarchy and even become the contrary of its expected outcome. I am one of those—an ally to the fight of women to cease gender-based disparities.

I was born in Saint-Louis, in northern Senegal, and grew up in Dakar until I was seven. When my parents decided to divorce (which I didn't know back then), my mother sent me and my little brother to Thiès (seventy kilometres from Dakar) at her brother's to protect us from their divorce. The stay, which was supposed to last for the duration of the divorce proceedings, ended up lasting eleven years. It was eleven years of physical suffering in a polygamous home (my uncle had three wives, two of whom lived under the same roof), in which anything could be a reason for a violent dispute or a fight between children of the same father but of different mothers. It was eleven years of struggle for even the most basic of things—a spot to sleep at night, a blanket during the cold winter, food, or clean clothes to put on—and to escape the beatings from the bigger ones who'd whoop your ass just because they could. It was eleven years in which—more so than the physical pain—the permanent emotional suffering as well as the unanswered questions of a child and later of an adolescent were the most difficult to deal with. I ended up forgetting my father, even his face. He didn't exist anymore. I was angry at my mother because she came to visit us regularly but only had a slight idea about the hardships my brother and I were going through. (Of course, every time she visited us, we were well treated for the duration of her visit.) I was furious at her every time she left to go back to Dakar without us; she would abandon us in that house to fear, bullying, beatings, and hunger. Then my little brother—who was epileptic, deaf, and dumb—died there. I did not utter a word the day when he died. I was sad and angry. I just cried silently, for a long time.

The death of my little brother did, however, give me the right that year to go on vacation to Dakar for a month. Beyond the joy of seeing again the place where I had always felt safe, I discovered the new life of my mother; she had rented a small room in the house of a young couple in Cité Marine. My mother had never been to school and never had a job. My father had been her second husband, and after their divorce, she remained single for almost ten years. She had decided to build herself a life, without depending on a man, free from the constraints of a marriage. My half-siblings (from her first marriage) were already grown, and some were already married or had a job. She told everyone that she wanted her independence. She wanted it for herself and to take care of my needs by herself. To do so, my mom had started a small business of selling various little products for women (fabrics, jewelry, incense, sheets, etc.), which she sold to her friends as well as others, and it worked pretty well. Being from Saint-Louis, she had always had that reputation of elegance and that of a woman of taste. She made a living from that small business for years and was able to take care of me. Coming back to Dakar every summer for holidays allowed me to realize how challenging life was to her but also how determined she was to depend solely on herself. She finally married again (probably because Senegalese traditions and Islam recommend that an adult woman should not remain unmarried), but she paid for the apartment she lived in with two of my divorced sisters and their children until she died in 1992. I was then twenty and decided to move back to Dakar definitely.

That segment of my mother's life, combined with the stories of my sisters (two of whom had had completely disastrous marriages with abusive husbands and another one, a teacher, whose home was more stable but had let several good professional opportunities escape simply because her husband, a teacher too, did not want her to earn more than him) opened my eyes to the intricacies of life as a woman within Senegalese society but especially to their lack of protection in spaces considered sacred, such as marriage. Indeed, in a society where we are told at an early age that there is nothing stronger or more meaningful than blood ties and family, why had it become so common to see women as well as their children physically or psychologically abused, and often without any assistance provided other than that of close family or friends? Why was I seeing all around me a multitude of children and teenagers with a history almost similar to mine? Like in my childhood, I saw absent as well as indifferent fathers. Like in my childhood, I saw mothers who had been made to believe that the greatest achievement of their life was to marry and create a family only to have that reality fall apart and be forced return to their parents' home with their children but without a job and often hope.

Growing up in that atmosphere and witnessing the pain of the women around me made me not want to be an unjust man—a man who would make children but not be involved in their life. I grew up telling myself that I would not be my father; I would not repeat his mistakes with my children. I promised myself to give my children all the attention and affection that my father hadn't given me. Of course, in hindsight, I smile at my naive resolutions because I have come to learn that building a life of fairness and decency is not as easy as one might think at a certain age. But I have learned that it is much more difficult to deconstruct modes of thought that have been legitimized by the society you have grown up in and whose manifestations are hidden in the most innocuous actions of our everyday life.

In 2008, I was in my mid-thirties and living in Dakar with Sandy, my German girlfriend, who I had been with for a year and a half. We'd just had a girl we named Asani (a Swahili name meaning "Rebellious"). She had come with the summer, on June 21, in Cologne. A few months earlier, we welcomed the news of Sandy's pregnancy with extreme happiness and excitement but did not have any discussion about how to educate or raise her. We were just sure that we wanted a baby, that we shared fundamental life principles, and that we wanted her to grow up in Dakar. For the rest, we were open to learning and adapting once our baby was born. The most important thing for me during her pregnancy was to be there for Sandy. In Dakar and Cologne, I went with her to several meetings with doctors as well as exercise classes for pregnant women. On the day of the delivery (by C-section), I went into the room with her. I still cannot describe what I felt in that moment. It must have been too overwhelming. I still remember everything, but the uniqueness of what I felt makes it impossible to put into words. I cried a lot, talked to Sandy, and tried to make her laugh. I stroked her head. Then, after some time, we heard the baby screaming.

Immediately after our return from Germany, Sandy resumed her work in a graphic design and photography agency. I had made the decision to put on hold most of my activities as a musician to take care of our daughter. For years, my work had made me travel a lot, but I declined any offer to leave Senegal for almost eighteen months after her birth. Sandy would go to work every day at 7:30 a.m. and return at 5:00 p.m., and I would spend the day with Asani. It went on like that for six months until we finally could afford a nanny. That period was important in my relationship with my daughter. Beyond the great intimacy that period created between the two of us, it helped my daughter grow up without any preconceived examples of gender roles in our house. Actually from the beginning of our life together in 2007, Sandy and I had naturally adopted that model, and I often was the one who cooked, did the dishes, and cleaned the house, whereas she had more skills related to repairing broken things in our house. All the time she was growing up, Asani has never experienced any activities done exclusively by one of us based on our gender. Except for breastfeeding, Sandy and I have equally done almost all activities with her. The same model still works, except for the things Asani can now do by herself.

We had created our own safe space, a bubble within which we did things according to our beliefs, and it worked as long as we were at home. The most difficult things were the external glances as well as the questions about our relationship, especially in a country where some things remained strongly anchored in gender stereotypes. Once, I was visiting a friend with my daughter who was barely a year old, his wife nearly choked when I wanted to change Asani's dirty diapers, arguing that it was not "a man's job." As for my sisters, they were always shocked by the fact that she was not braided but instead had an afro which made her "look less like a girl." Why doesn't she wear dresses? Why isn't she having earrings? There were questions, a lot of questions. All of that was accompanied by advice on an assortment of topics, including my responsibility to set a good example for her to grow up as a good Muslim and to make sure that she speaks Wolof, my mother tongue. But rather than being annoyed, I would discuss our choices with them, joke about it, but remain firm in our decision to raise our daughter in our own way. I'm not sure I've always been understood, but my goal was to make it clear to my family and friends that we wanted our child to have a fair balance of the two cultures she originated from and to give her the possibility of experiencing the best of both worlds.

Asani is growing up fast. She is ten years old. Sandy and I separated when she was seven—a separation that happened without too much drama because we both agreed that we had to preserve our daughter as best we could. We sat down together to explain to her that dad was going to leave, that she would now have two homes in Dakar, but that our love for her hadn't changed and would never change. Of course, she refused to understand or to accept it. Maintaining the dialogue between Sandy and me, while avoiding any of the heavier discussions in her presence, allowed her to see that we were not tearing apart and that there was still this bond of mutual respect she had been growing in for seven years. Even though it was difficult to witness, we accepted the expression of her incomprehension and anger, and it helped us all to trust her intelligence, talk to her, and explain, to the extent that it was possible, the new situation we were in and that we would keep taking care of her but in two different homes.

On Saturday, March 31, 2018 I spent the day with Asani today. We went to the bookstore before eating in the gardens of the French Institute of Dakar where we stayed to do colouring until mid-afternoon. Then at 5:00 p.m., we proceeded to the movies to see Ava Duvarnay's *A Wrinkle in Time* before I took her back to her mom's. We also took the opportunity to discuss a punishment she had had from her mom that week for secretly using her tablet when she's only allowed to use it during the weekends. Her mom had told me about it on the phone, and Asani cried, recognized her wrongdoing, but still defending herself. In the end, she promised to talk to her mother again and to apologize again—a little episode that sums up pretty well my relationship with my daughter, since we are not living together anymore. We talk almost every day on the phone—discussing school, friends, her sports, or arts activities—and spend our weekends together. Despite the frustration of not seeing each other every day, we have an amazing relationship. Sandy and I have never been before a judge to decide anything about Asani. We have agreed in an amicable and a reasonable way that it would be best—because my job requires me to travel a lot—that Asani stays with her during the week and I take her during the weekends. I now realize, despite the failure of my childhood dream of a strong and united family, that it is possible to be a parent for your child even if you do not live together. I am involved in my daughter's life; I go to each of her school shows, attend parents' meetings with her mother when I'm in Dakar, and equally pay for all the expenses related to her life. When friends congratulate me sometimes for doing all of those things for my daughter, I laugh and realize how much the norm has been misled. I do not deserve any medals for just doing my fair share of parenting responsibilities. You do not congratulate a father on acting like a father. And very often my daughter is the first to remind me of that. On several occasions, when I'm too lazy to cook for example, she often says to me jokingly, "You're the daddy, so do what you have to do!" To hear that sentence, out of my child's mouth, makes me face my responsibilities, even those beyond cooking her something to eat.

Listening to my daughter is what ultimately characterizes my relationship with her today. Over time, I have come to understand that being a father to her means to acknowledge her opinion, desires, and feelings, and not to decide unilaterally for her or even for me when it has consequences for her. Once, two years ago, I was out with her to buy her new shoes and without realizing it, I was trying to convince her to take a pair of Converses that I found cute but she did not like. At one point, she said, "I've seen shoes that I like, but I'm sure you're going to say no." I was taken aback and replied, "But ... why do you think that I will say no?" "Because you say no to everything I say," she said. I was ashamed of myself but proud that she spoke her mind. We had finally returned home with the shoes she wanted and that I did not like at all, but it made me think about the limits I had to have as a parent and not to interfere in things as personal as the colour or patterns of her clothes or other accessories. Since then, I've been careful not to repeat the same mistake.

We discuss everything. No subject is considered too serious for her or too childish for me. It's just a matter of finding the right words, or for some practical things or questions that I do not have answers to, we ask Google. As an adult, I perceive the effect that such an approach has on her personality. Although she is reserved by nature, Asani also has great self-confidence, expresses herself, and has a great sense of responsibility. Throughout our interactions, I am learning a lot about being a father and about me. I learn by observing and listening to the criticisms Asani often makes about my decisions and my ways of doing things. Since her birth, I have sure questioned many of my adult certainties.

The other important aspect of my relationship with my daughter is the fact that she is a girl. It is obviously important that she is aware of her gender and that she feels comfortable in her body and identity, but since her birth, the fact that she is a girl has never had a major influence on how we are raising her. As I said earlier, we really do discuss everything, and we do talk about such issues as difference, discrimination, race, and religion. That is my way to not keep her in a bubble and to help her prepare for a world that she's already confronted with but can't always decipher all of its subtleties. I told her that many will want to define her, limit her, and will have expectations from her simply based on her gender. She did not understand at first, probably because the gender issue was not prevalent in the family setting in which she grew up. But her school taught her about gender when she was told by the boys that she could not play football with them because she was a girl. Some of the girls in the school eventually created their own team, and they now regularly play against the boys. At home, for house chores, I encourage her to help me and teach her how to do certain things, but always with the idea to make her more independent. I tried this approach with cooking, for example, but I always end up being the only one who prepares the meals.

Then there is the relationship to her body. As I implied earlier, it is important for me to protect my daughter, but it is more important to give her the means to protect herself, even at her age. When she started kindergarten at age three, her mother and I asked her to let us know if anyone ever touched her inappropriately. Then when she was four years old, I explained to her that I was going to stop helping her clean herself every time she went to the bathroom, which was meant to push her to learn to take care of her own cleanliness. But it was also an opportunity for her to ask questions and for me to explain a little about intimacy and how her body belongs to her. I think those notions are now firmly established within her, and it makes me smile when she now chases me out of the room whenever she is at home and has to change herself. Asani will soon be a teenager and will undergo significant transformations, physical ones among others. I hope that the consciousness she has of her body will keep growing and help her through her future puberty.

My mother started my education, and my daughter continues it, yet the two never met. Their times are different, but the challenges they face are almost similar, as they have both showed me why and how to treat a human being with respect and to be a decent man. My mother fought alone, but Asani will have me by her side. Although I will never be able to grasp the magnitude of what being a woman in this world means, I am sure to be an ally in their fight; I wish to see the cycle broken. Remembering my innumerable nights of sadness when I thought of my mother who was far from me and fighting for her dignity, I have no choice but to raise my child with love and protection and to prepare her for a world that will surely be hostile to her in many ways, including her gender. I am not idealizing things, but I am convinced that in order for definite change to happen regarding gender equality, it is important to start within our families and our children, boys and girls; it is important to recreate the balance there and teach them ways to be fair individuals. My journey with Asani is hopefully not over yet; adolescence is coming, and I am sure I will learn more from her, and she will learn more from me, too. Either way, one thing is certain: I will always walk with my daughter.

Chapter 25

Feminists Opened My Eyes

Oliver Ngweno

I am twenty years old. I know that my parents and role models have most likely already influenced me to a great degree, but I haven't determined my part in society yet. Without knowing my role in society, it is difficult to determine the significance of other people's influence on my actions, as I simply haven't acted yet.

Nevertheless, I am an opinionated person. For as much as I have agency over my own life, I believe that my view of our societies, as well as their merits and faults, shall determine the choices I make and the roles I will play in the future. I must credit the feminists in my life for leading me to believe that women deserve the equality that they don't have yet in the modern world.

My mother is a single parent, and I'm an only child, so it's hard for me to state what feminist parenting is. I knew nothing different. My mother, in her career, has managed to change the lives of thousands of people through humanitarian work and has created and promoted technologies to help advance the developing world. Growing up with such a well-informed parent, the statements I made that began with "My mother told me..." were more likely to be fact than fiction. Whenever my aunt, who has a PhD, visited, I would listen to her discussions with my mother and grandmother. After growing up with such intelligent women, I find it astonishing that many people still disregard women's opinions because of gender-based prejudices. These were the people that raised me. They opened my eyes to sexism in all the fields in which I worked.

Growing up in Kenya, gender stereotyping was common, but I had no shortage of female role models. My mother, my aunt, and my grandmother were strong characters in the family and also publicly known in their professional lives. When I decided to become serious about playing tennis at the age of thirteen, my tennis coach was a woman, and when I graduated from that level, the Kenya national coach was also a woman. Under their guidance, I've learned how to be competitive, disciplined, goal oriented, and focused. When I look back at how these women have contributed to the person I am becoming, I think they combine strength with empathy in a way that may not be as easy for men.

Comprehending gender inequality around me is challenging because it is so entwined with other aspects of culture. It would be impossible to discuss my experiences regarding gender roles without considering ethnicity, national identity, and religion. Sometimes I played the stereotypes to my advantage. For example, I always had pink covers for my phones because I knew the boys at school would never "borrow" them.

By the time I was thirteen years old, I started travelling around eastern and southern Africa to participate in international competitions. I had also lived in the U.S. for four years. Because of these travels and absences, I am sometimes viewed as an outsider in my home country, which makes it difficult for people to consider my perspectives. They immediately dismiss them as foreign and, therefore, invalid. The problem I face is that it has become difficult to counter blatant sexism. On one occasion, I found myself in a conversation with a group of young men, who had unanimously agreed that all women were subordinate to all men. It was amazing to me that in 2018, young men with whom I had grown up could actually hold this opinion.

As soon as I began to question their statements, I was accused of having been misled by foreign skeptics into disbelieving God. According to their logic, God is male, and God created man in his image, and it is, therefore, man's right to be superior to woman. I realized I wasn't going to convince them otherwise. I felt disappointed and defeated. What concerned me even more was that these men are yet to be married or have children. The greatest effect of their prejudice is yet to be felt.

A few days later, I was approached by one of the men again. He was determined to prove God's masculinity to me, this time, in the presence of a twelve-year-old girl. Determined to shame me, he loudly accused me of disobeying the Bible for proposing that God might not have a gender. He turned to the girl and said that leaders are male, hence the head of your household is male and so is God. In a single stark remark, the girl replied, "My father is not God!"

Although my concern that my generation is continuing a culture of prejudice and intolerance persists, my hope was renewed by the girl. Despite being a child and female in an environment dominated by adult males, she expressed her opinion confidently and defiantly. Thankfully, now more than ever, children have greater freedom to express themselves, which allows them to take small steps away from oppression and prejudice.

Another lesson for me is that children aren't solely a product of how their parents raise them. They have minds of their own. In the same way the girl refused to accept that she is a lesser member of society, a child can be defiant when told to be kind or generous. For better or for worse, parents have less control of their children than they may like to think. I believe that all we can do is encourage our children to appreciate diversity and teach them to be expressive in situations they find unfair.

Unfortunately, in my experience, not everyone wants equality. There are still people out there who constantly belittle others. So far, it has been impossible for me to convince people that sexism is harmful to society. They believe they are right and that they have the right to feel and act superior and dominate others. The only person we can change is ourselves. But just as my feminist mother and feminist role models in my life opened my eyes, I hope my commitment to equality between the sexes may, in turn, open the eyes of others.

Day after day, I try to make a difference. So far, the only changes I have witnessed would have happened on their own. Today, I am tired of trying, but my mother taught me to be persistent, so tonight I will rest, and tomorrow, perhaps, I will succeed.

Chapter 26

The Struggling Feminists

Ousmane Diop

> "Of course I am not worried about intimidating men. The type of man who will be intimidated by me is exactly the type of man I have no interest in."
>
> —*Chimamanda Ngozi Adichie (qtd. in Goyal 72)*

Expecting our first child raises many questions that should not be taken for granted. Financial readiness is crucial; it is, however, not the most important factor. An understanding of the relationship between culture, socioeconomic factors, and worldviews are necessary alongside emotional support and guidance throughout the child's formative years. But for someone like me who defines myself as feminist, it is also important to explore gender roles within my environment and decide the aspects of different cultures with which I want to nurture my boy. This process is not easy; it is a constant battle with different fringes of society and with oneself. At the end of the day, I want my son (and my daughter, if we have one) to experience true equal opportunity—one where boys are allowed to cry without shame, and girls do not experience any form of glass ceiling in pursing their dreams.

I uttered my first word and kicked my first ball in Senegal, the most western point of the African continent. Senegal is a country where roles and responsibilities within the family are still very gendered—men still mostly provide the livelihood, and women still bring up children and manage the household. These roles were even more segregated when I was a child back in the eighties; it was common to say that the kitchen was a women-only zone, in which men were not allowed. I remember being told by my female cousins to leave the kitchen to avoid bad luck. In over thirty years, things have changed for the better with the introduction of parity laws in the political arena, for instance. However, although it's important to recognize the significance of this and the opportunity that it offers women in Senegal, so long as men are still allowed up to four wives and are still deemed the head of the family, we cannot talk about real gender equality in Senegalese society.

My family was a little different from the typical family in my neighbourhood. Even though my mum stayed home to look after the seven of us and told me things like "boys do not cry," she would also ask my brothers and me to sweep the floor or do the washing up after we finished eating. Whether this was a deliberate attempt to be fairer to my sisters—or a plan to prepare us for a changing world where household chores would be shared between partners—it certainly made me uncomfortable when my friends found me doing "women's work" at home. Nevertheless, it planted within me the first seeds of feminism, as it made me compare my situation with my friends' and question the status quo of gender roles. During arguments, older friends would just laugh at me, as if to say: "one day you'll understand," whereas my peers or younger friends would start quoting the Qur'an or the Prophetic Sunnah. I cannot recollect the number of times I have been asked the question "Do you believe in the Qur'an or not?" It was an attempt to stop me from challenging practices that are permitted in Islam by making me choose between my religion and personal beliefs.

Growing up, I considered myself a fair person who would challenge gender inequalities when I saw them. I saw myself as a champion of women's rights—until I met my girlfriend (now wife), who challenged many more of my unquestioned views and referred me to authors I had never heard of. She asked me simple questions that no one had asked me before: "Why do children automatically take their father's last name in both of our societies?" or "Why don't men cook even when both partners are working?" or "Why will you not call yourself feminist?" Even though the questions were simple, I did not have convincing answers for her. And although I was happy to challenge the status quo at times, I was not comfortable carrying the "feminist" label until the early 2010s. Some might argue that I feared the association with the word. Others might see a slow process of reeducation. Ultimately, I have reached a point in my thinking where I can comfortably say that I am a feminist, and I try to live by standards of true equality between men and women, which is one of my best definitions of the concept.

Challenging my ideas and ways of life was the first step in my personal reeducation; the second step was establishing exactly what kind of feminism I identified with. I thought about whether issues came down to societal structures or individual agency and whether I thought the problem was solely men and their hunger for power or was it a societal problem, including men and women. These are questions and ideas we discuss. I am still undecided on many issues. I am somewhere in the middle. In the meantime, I have to live with my partner, and we need to find ways of putting feminism into practice for us. We need to make it a reality. Our feminism must be beyond all the literature and schools of thought, and it must allow room for our backgrounds, experiences, and life stories.

I left my native Senegal at the age of twenty-seven, and everything suddenly changed. I left the comfort of my family for a life of flat sharing with my girlfriend and two of her friends, Hazel and Camille. I met Hazel in Senegal when she had come to work as language assistant in Dakar; I did not know Camille, but I was told that we had a few things in common, including the fact that we were both francophones and anglophiles. I remember flying to London hoping that those two would be enough to create a rapport and a good basis to live together in our Stoke Newington flat. Learning to live with new people in a totally new environment was not easy, but the biggest challenge I faced was taking responsibility for a fair amount of household chores. When I arrived in London in October 2008, I knew how to cook basic meals, such as omelettes and spaghetti. I had never used a washing machine before, nor had I been expected to cook and clear up 50 per cent of the time.

This was going to be my new life—a life where we shared all chores equally. This was a big change for me. I had to fight against myself and the unequal treatment of women I had absorbed. I had to challenge society and what it had taught me from the day I was born. I was finally becoming a feminist—one that decided to step outside of patriarchy and help free people from that system as well as one that started to put the theory, or at least parts of the theory, into practice. I can still remember my first experience shopping at Tesco with my girlfriend as well as the first meal I cooked for the two of us. These were great achievements and important steps towards equality in our relationship.

Of course, the practice is not as straightforward as the theory wants it to be. When life becomes busy and time scarce, one tends to go back to what one knows and to what is comfortable and easy. In my case, this consisted of looking after the garden and repairing electrical issues around the flat. As for my partner, she often takes on the role of managing household chores, planning our next holiday, and managing our social diary. Indeed, when too much is going on and we do not have time and energy for an argument, it becomes easier for me to repair the lamp than to wait for her to do it, and it would be easier for her to organize the next social gathering than to leave it with me. Whether this is just a failure to practice what we preach or a normal phase in the long and winding journey to self-reeducation, we must accept that it is a constant battle—a battle with ourselves and with the world around us.

My wife and I are struggling feminists. We discuss feminism a great deal. We love to explore the various theories with friends. We compare childhood experiences and current ideas and thoughts. We are, however, far from being perfect feminists. Our feminist relationship is a work in progress. We support each other's feminism and continue to challenge each other's gendered roles at times. We learn from each other as we continue in this journey, and we always hope to do things better next time. This is not different from other areas of life—an ever-changing environment with new lessons and new actors all the time. In our case, the next actor was our new son; he was born at the end of December 2017. The question that remains is how two struggling feminists will bring up a child as a feminist.

I believe that children are born like a blank canvas waiting to be drawn on. They do not have any idea of racism, sexism or homophobia. Their family, school, and the people they meet and spend time with will play a significant role in shaping the kinds of views that the child will hold and the behaviours they will develop. I once was that child, and I remember asking myself all kinds of questions at the time my wife was pregnant. Financially, we were ready to welcome a third person into our family, but there is more to bringing up a child than financial readiness. It is our responsibility to make sure we pass on our experiences and values to him, which, of course, include gender equality and mutual respect. We want to raise him as a true feminist. We will have to share our understanding of the lines between our cultures and our worldviews.

We will have to provide emotional support and guidance to him throughout his formative years.

Our son will grow up with various expectations. On the one hand, he will be expected to respect women and girls as true equals and not to participate in oppression. On the other, as a mixed-race child growing up in Britain, he will inevitably experience some racism. This means he will have to let go of certain privileges given to him on account of being male while also learning to assert himself and claiming other privileges that will be taken from him for not being white. Feminism is at its most interesting when it is intersectional (Crenshaw) and takes into account other factors of inequality, such as race, class, or ability. Indeed, as women from different backgrounds experience varying kinds of patriarchal expectations and oppressions, women sometimes find aspects of their identities brought into conflict or their disadvantages ignored by members of the dominant group. Our son will have to weigh up the privileges and disadvantages of differing aspects of his identity and understand the nuances of situations where they come into play in order to make good decisions throughout his life.

Our relationship as a couple had changed when we were expecting our son. Space had been created organically into which to welcome the baby. That space had been growing as we got closer to the due date, as we focused more and more on baby-related matters and the planning of life after his arrival. Our relationship with friends and family had also changed as we shared our plans with them. We found it difficult to talk about anything other than baby-related subjects and answering questions around raising a mixed-race child, raising a child with two languages, and, of course, raising a child as a feminist. One recurrent theme has been what names our child would have.

I believe that the name one gives one's child should be meaningful. It must be traced back to one's family, cultural, or political influences, among others. As for my wife, she has been focusing more on names she likes right now. I wanted us to choose a name that had a resonance for either or both of us. We finally managed to agree after months of discussions. The process to choosing a family name was even longer, with various considerations: the double barrel option, the middle-name option, or the newly created name option. We finally opted for the double barrel to acknowledge both of our families and cultures. I hope our son will have the opportunity to fully experience both cultures and will be able to pick and choose the most positive aspects while leaving behind the negative in both of our cultures.

The journey so far has been long, interesting, and challenging. But an even more interesting one has now started with the arrival of our first child. My wife and I have been able to shed many patriarchal aspects of both our cultures, and we want to continue learning as we share experiences with him. I am aware that I will not be able to raise the perfect feminist, partly because I am not a perfect one but also because he will explore different environments and meet people I have no control over. But I shall be content if my son grows up believing that boys can actually cry, that they can feel and express a range of emotions, and that feminine is not a synonym of weak. I also want him to truly respect women through reading their writing and having women among his role models while growing up. I will teach him fairness at home by continuing to do my part of the workload around the flat. Furthermore, I will endeavour to make sure my son is strong enough to speak up and call out other people when they have been sexist. Finally, I want him to understand the meaning of "no means no" so that he will always hear and respect women's boundaries.

I want our son (and our daughter, if we have one) to experience only real equal opportunity in Britain, Senegal, or anywhere else we decide to live. I want to help create a society where boys can cry without shame and one where girls can expect to earn the same salary as their male counterparts, a society where I do not have to convince my brother to opt out of polygamy when he gets married, a society where politicians are fifty-fifty male and female, and equality is central in all policymaking, a society where I do not have to feel strange asking for a longer paternity leave than my male colleagues, and a society where all of its members focus on dismantling the structural barriers to equality so that feminism does not remain only an individual issue.

Works Cited

Crenshaw, Kimberlé. "Mapping the Margins: Intersectionality, Identity Politics, and Violence against Women of Color." *Racial Equality Tools*, 1991, www.racialequitytools.org/resourcefiles/mapping-margins.pdf. Accessed 19 Feb. 2020.

Goyal, Nehaa. *UGC NET JRF Women's Studies Paperback*. Educreation Publishing, 2018.

Chapter 27

"Work Hard for Your Little Girl" and Other Dilemmas of Feminist Tightrope Walkers

Alioune 'Papa'

Welcoming my daughter into the world back in October 2016 was the greatest gift I have ever received in life. As I held my love in my hands while she was looking into my eyes with so much attention, my heart melted. She was so fragile, so fearless and so innocent, but the moment was promptly interrupted! Very soon, my happiness met with anxiety. She was welcomed into a world where she will face a number of challenges as a girl and woman. The way we, as parents, educate and influence her will predominantly shape her future.

This chapter discusses my initiation to parenthood and attempts to understand the man I am today, including my definition of feminism and how I apply it to my everyday life. As a young and first-time parent, my experiences as a child, teenager, now adult have contributed to how I make the choices I do today.

As a Child and Teenager

From a modest background, I have violently but silently resisted the idea that men have more professional duties, whereas domestic duties, such as cooking and raising children, belong to women. I say "silently" because my family was as patriarchal as the other families around us. I grew up and evolved in two contrasting environments: from boyhood to my early adolescence and from adolescence to my young adulthood.

I spent my first twelve years in Senegal; my dad was the breadwinner, whereas my mother stayed at home and took care of my other six siblings and me. As I was close to my mother, I saw how much of a brilliant professional career she could have had if she had been allowed to pursue her passions. Yet my father and mother did not challenge the established gender roles of our traditional Senegalese culture. At a very young age, I could not stand seeing my mother doing all the household work without any help from my father. As boys, we were also raised not to help with household chores. And growing up in Senegal, where gender norms are highly accentuated, my sister and I were most of the time supporting my mother with these responsibilities. At best, I created strategies to assist my mother as much as I could. I remember often playing a game with friends in my home, asking them to spill soapy water on the floor and inviting them to show their best gliding movements. After this little game, I would usually give a floor cloth to each one to contribute to the cleaning. I guess this was also my way of challenging the gendered behaviour of boys.

At the age of thirteen, I moved in with my Senegalese uncle and his French wife in France. In my new home, I lived with three cousins, whom I considered my siblings: two white female cousins from a previous marriage, one older than me by two years, the other younger by three; and one very young, mixed-heritage son of my aunt and uncle, who got married two years prior to my arrival and recreated this wonderful stepfamily. Roles, then, were a lot more gender balanced because both my uncle and aunt were working fulltime, and at home, they shared the household management. The word "feminism" never entered my mind and was never pronounced at home, but I was witnessing true partnership in the house. They would share and debate how best to raise children without gender stereotyping them. Or they would together discuss the costs related to running the household, among other matters. This experience shaped my views and instilled within me true egalitarian values.

As an Adult

Yet today, in my early thirties, I am still exploring my political, socioeconomic, and cultural views as to understanding the complexity of feminism in all its varieties in order to establish a definition of feminism that I am comfortable with. However, I would not use the label "feminist" to define myself. My feminism is one that treats both men and women equally in all spheres of life and is attentive to issues of justice. I would identify as an ally rather than a feminist, as I am still learning what feminism means for me.

Becoming a Dad and Thriving for Greater Professional Autonomy and Financial Sustainability

Of the many concerns I had upon the birth of my daughter, financial stability was the one that most loudly resonated in my head. Eight months before her birth, I woke up early in the morning and very anxiously typed a note on my smartphone set at 6:00 a.m. as a daily memo. Today, nearly two years later, the notification still shows up in the morning: "Work hard for your little girl." I knew her sex before she was born, despite my wife's strong belief it would be a boy. I guess paternal instinct does exist. Earning enough money for my family's needs in the United Kingdom and in Senegal remains important, but I make sure not to forget the most essential things in life: ensuring the needs of my daughter, being a positive influence for her, and instilling important values within her.

I am blessed that I was able to work part time when my daughter was born, as this allowed me to enjoy my parental leave and spend time with her. Yet I regret being unable to fully support my wife in her fieldwork study. We also face many challenges in dividing family roles in an equal fashion. I believe this will be the greatest challenge my daughter confronts—a society organized around strict and sometimes oppressive gender roles.

Like Tightrope Walkers

Although we still face numerous challenges in the equal division of our roles, especially while our baby is still breastfeeding, we are more able to achieve a balance since our daughter has attended nursery school part time, and my wife can do her research. Every day, we challenge the gendered social constructs of the households we knew growing up. Above all, as a father to my daughter, I have a crucial role to play in defying established norms and roles, particularly as they relate to parenting both in our inner circle and in society at large. I truly believe that gender equality will only come with the elimination of gendered parenting roles and behaviour. I constantly ask myself where to start and whether I do enough. I am doing my best to be present in all spheres of my family life in order to transmit egalitarian values to my daughter.

I think it is essential that our daughter grows up aware of gendered discrimination and injustice so that she is equipped to challenge them. I will encourage her to be self-assured and entitled to all that she works hard for and to resist racism and sexism in all of their manifestations. I will support her as she breaks the glass ceiling and smashes patriarchy. I want her to be the strongest and most opinioned person in the room, but I want her to be able to defend her views while listening to her interlocutors' points of view and to have the capacity to admit when she is wrong. I seek to support my wife and daughter as well as the women in my life as a feminist ally. This adventure makes me think of us as tightrope walkers. I am their ally who will support them as we walk the tightrope across and over patriarchy.

Chapter 28

Lessons on Feminist Parenting from My Nonfeminist Mother

Françoise Kpeglo Moudouthe

My mother never claimed to be a feminist, yet I became a feminist because of her. My feminist journey started on a hot morning in Douala, when I was about five years old. Tired of hearing me moan about having to go to school again, my mother stooped down and looked me right in the eye—a sign that things were about to get serious. She whispered: "You're going to school today and every day after that. And once you're there, you will focus and do your best. That's how you will make your own money, so that if a man ever tries to throw you out of his house, you can tell him to leave because it's your house, too."

I will never forget the fire in her eyes. She had that same resolute look I would glimpse from the backseat every morning as she put her car's makeup mirror to good use, carefully applying her lipstick as if she hadn't just said we were running late. The urgency in her voice would become a familiar tune in the soundtrack of my childhood. I would hear it every time she pointed out that I hadn't earned any of the privileges I was enjoying as a child, and she instructed me to direct my prayers and actions to support less fortunate children like my cousins, neighbours, and the children in the orphanage where she volunteered her time.

By the time I started calling myself a feminist, I was convinced that my mother was one too—until I wasn't. The marriage advice she gave me on the eve of my wedding was surprisingly conservative. She became increasingly vocal about her disapproval of other young women's choices while she chose to remain silent in the face of injustices these same women were submitted to.

Within a few years my disbelief grew into disappointment, which, I'm now ashamed to admit, translated into cutting remarks I hope she will forgive one day. Let's just say that if there is a special place in hell for daughters who are unfair to their mothers, and that's probably where I will be spending my afterlife.

When I finally mustered the courage to ask her what had made her turn away from feminism, she replied, "Did I ever tell you I was a feminist?" A few seconds later, she added, "Life happened." I instantly knew what she meant. It's a long story, as you can imagine, and it's not mine to tell. So today I will share not my mother's life story but what I have learned from her about feminist parenting.

"Life Happened"

With just two words, my mother taught me to let go of the idea that the only way I could earn the right to call myself a feminist parent was if I managed to embody my feminist values perfectly and at all times.

I no longer blame myself for feeling a hint of shame every time I utter the word "vulva" in front of my daughter. Instead, I celebrate myself for not passing that shame on to her. I no longer panic at the idea that over the years, my feminist principles may waver in the face of the kind of pain and disillusions my mother had to face—and that I might confuse my children with my mixed messages. I simply make sure they are imbibing enough feminist values from me every day so that they don't let any turns in their mother's journey affect their own.

I had always thought of feminist parenting as a battle against the patriarchal messages that hide in textbooks, schoolyards and cartoons. My mother taught me to also watch out for the enemy within. I now know I must reject my own obsession with perfection and just show up for my daughter and my son as well as I can on any given day. As my children grow, they learn from me even before I feel worthy of teaching them. Teaching my daughter to cherish her body doesn't have to wait until I am able to wipe off the disgust that still lingers on my face whenever I look at my belly fat rolls in the mirror. Life does happen, and so I will keep doing my best until I can do better.

I grew up hearing that "impossible is not Cameroonian," as people say on the streets of Douala. Shifting the focus of my feminist parenting from achieving perfection to imparting incomplete knowledge has, therefore, been more arduous than I would have liked. Thanks to my mother, I have learned the importance of prioritizing the messages I want my children to take in as they grow up.

My mother had focused on raising her daughters to become independent women and empathetic human beings. I have decided to put freedom at the heart of my feminist parenting. I want both my daughter and my son to be free to be who they want to be. I want them to speak up without the fear of stigma and silence that still keeps me silent sometimes.

Being a mother undoubtedly motivates me to be a better feminist. What I have learned from my mother is that I am in no position to judge another mother—and certainly not mine—for doing the best she could with what she had.

Most importantly, I have learned that feminist parenting doesn't afford me with the luxury of sequencing the feministing and the parenting. I now know that I don't have to become a perfect feminist to raise powerful ones.

Afterword

Trajectories and Topographies of Feminist Parenting: Established Routes and New Pathways

Andrea O'Reilly

The concept of feminist mothering is drawn from the important distinction Rich makes in *Of Woman Born: Motherhood as Experience and Institution* between two meanings of motherhood, one superimposed on the other: "the potential relationship of any woman to her powers of reproduction and to children," and "the institution—which aims at ensuring that that potential and all women —shall remain under male control" (13). The term "motherhood," thus, refers to the patriarchal institution of motherhood, which is male defined and controlled and oppressive to women, whereas the word "mothering" refers to women's experiences of mothering, which are female defined and potentially empowering to women. This distinction enabled feminist scholars to view motherhood as not naturally, necessarily, or inevitably oppressive; on the contrary, mothering, freed from motherhood, may be experienced as a site of empowerment and as a location of social change if, to use Rich's words, women became "outlaws from the institution of motherhood" (195).

Although much has been published on patriarchal motherhood since Rich's inaugural text—research that documents why and how patriarchal motherhood is harmful, indeed unnatural, to mothers and children alike—the topic of feminist mothering has only recently received robust issues, Green identifies four commons themes in the interviews: participants understand motherhood to be an institution and experience; they consciously mother as feminists; they practice elements of feminist pedagogy; and they engage in feminist praxis while mothering. (76) For me, the most illuminating and instructive concept that emerges from Green's study can be termed the "dialectical and transformative nature of feminist mothering" (76).

Feminist theorists, as Green writes, "have established an inherent contradiction in motherhood; while motherhood is strongly associated with access to an internalization of patriarchal power, it simultaneously is a place where women can create their own mothering strategies to challenge various dominant power strategies" (57). Significantly, the mothers of Green's study, in language and tone evocatively similar to those of Adrienne Rich, speak passionately and often about this contradiction. The mothers make visible what is often invisible about institutionalized motherhood: they acknowledge the confining aspects of motherhood; recognize how regulatory elements of the institution are harmful to women and children; and speak to the low self-esteem, self-blame, and self-hatred of internalized oppression. However, as the women identify and catalogue the many ways that motherhood is an oppressive and a repressive institution, they, in and through this critique, "create some distance from it and make space within mothering to mother in ways that are suitable to them" and, in so doing, "engage in a self-reflexive creating of subjectivity to redefine motherhood for themselves" (84). Such transformative practices include the following: mothering outside of heterosexual relationships; living apart from the father and mothering alone; rejecting the wife role expected of mothers; renouncing the belief that mothers are totally responsible for the character of the child; challenging the assumption that mothers will raise their children according to patriarchal expectations; developing feminist styles of childrearing; creating other models for family; and practicing nonauthoritative ways of parenting. When defined on its own terms, mothering becomes, to borrow from Green, "a dynamic place for creativity" (113). What Green's study shows is that patriarchal motherhood is neither completely oppressive nor nonnegotiable. In it, mothers do find room to practice agency, resistance, and renewal. In this, the women's stories and Green's study realize the hope that Rich spoke to more than forty years ago—mothers have "managed to salvage for

[them]selves [and] for [their] children, even within the destructiveness of the institution ... the tenderness, the passion, the trust in our instincts, the evocation of a courage we did not know we owned" (280).

Green's book reveals that feminist mothers "are challenging motherhood, creating alternatives in mothering that transform the lives of mothers and of children and changing the meaning of both mothering and feminism" (4). Reading Green's book, I am reminded of Maureen Reddy's *Everyday Acts against Racism*, in which she explains that she chose the phrase "everyday acts" as her title to "emphasize the daily, the ordinary, as opposed to extraordinary" dimensions of antiracist parenting (ix). She concludes her introduction citing political scientist Howard Zinn: "When changes take place in history, they are not the result of a few heroic deeds, but of small actions—all that persistence creates a great social movement" (qtd. in Reddy xiii). What Green's work shows, or perhaps more appropriately teaches, to paraphrase Zinn, is that the politic, praxis, and pedagogy of feminist mothering, while expressed as everyday acts, are indeed the heroic deeds of a great social movement.

In my research on feminist mothering I explore how motherhood, as it is currently perceived and practiced in patriarchal societies, is disempowering if not oppressive for a multitude of reasons: namely, the societal devaluation of motherwork, the endless tasks of privatized mothering, and the impossible standards of idealized motherhood. My research seeks to identify the central themes and characteristics of feminist mothering. In the first instance, feminist mothering functions as an oppositional discourse of motherhood; more specifically, it signifies a theory and practice of mothering that seeks to challenge the dominant discourse of motherhood and change the various ways that the lived experience of patriarchal motherhood is limiting or oppressive to women. Most pointedly, I argue, the overarching aim of empowered mothering is to confer to mothers the agency, authority, authenticity, autonomy, and advocacy-activism denied to them in patriarchal motherhood. Maternal agency, as Lynn O'Brien Hallstein explains in her encyclopedia entry on the topic "draws on the idea of agency—the ability to influence one's life, to have a power to control one's life—and explores how women have agency via mothering (697)." A theory of maternal agency focuses on, as O'Brien Hallstein continues, "mothering practices that facilitate women's authority and power and is revealed in mothers' efforts to challenge and act against aspects of institutionalized motherhood that constrain and limit women's lives and power as mothers" (697). Inauthenticity, as explained in Elizabeth Butterfield's encyclopedia entry, "is an ethical term that denotes being true to oneself, as in making decisions that are consistent with one's own beliefs and values. In contrast, inauthenticity is generally understood to be an abdication of one's own authority and a loss of integrity (700). In the context of feminist mothering, maternal authenticity draws upon Ruddick's concept of the "conscientious mother" (1989) and my model of the "authentic feminist mother" (*Maternal Thinking*), and it refers to "independence of mind and the courage to stand up to dominant values" and to "being truthful about motherhood and remaining true to oneself" in motherhood" (Butterfield; 700; O'Reilly, "Between the Baby and the Bathwater). Similarly, maternal authority and autonomy refer to confidence and conviction in oneself—holding power in the household and the ability to define and determine one's life and practices of mothering and means the refusal to, in Ruddick's words, "relinquish or repudiate one's own perceptions and values" (112). Finally, the topic of maternal advocacy-activism foregrounds the political and social dimension of motherwork, whether such is expressed in antisexist childrearing or maternal activism. I also demarcate the defining characteristics of feminist mothering organized under the themes of motherhood, family, childrearing, and activism (O'Reilly, *Feminist Mothering*).

Central to all four attributes of feminist mothering is a redefinition of motherhood from a feminist-maternal perspective. Under the theme of motherhood, theorists of empowered mothering counter the normative discourse of motherhood as limited to middle-class, married, stay at-home moms to include a multitude of maternal identities—such as noncustodial, poor, single, young, old, and working mothers— and a variety of motherhood practices, such as the practices of other-mothering found in African-American culture and the comothering of queer households. Likewise, as the normative family is restricted to a patriarchal nuclear structure wherein the parents are married, and the mother is the nurturer and the father is the provider, the family formations of empowered mothers are many and varied to embrace single, blended, step, matrifocal, same sex, and so forth. Furthermore, although patriarchal motherhood characterizes childrearing as a private, nonpolitical undertaking, feminist mothering, concerned with the final two themes of childrearing and activism, builds upon the work of Sara Ruddick to redefine motherwork as a socially engaged enterprise and a site of power, wherein mothers can affect social change both in the home through feminist childrearing and outside the home through maternal activism. Feminist mothering foregrounds the political and social dimension of childrearing to emphasize how traditional practices of gender socialization may be challenged and corrected in antisexist childrearing practices to raise empowered daughters and empathetic sons. While those interested in activism examine how mothers may use their position to lobby for social and political change (Hill; Stadtman; Tucker; Powell; Nathanson; Kinser).

The current scholarship on feminist mothering, which was developed in response to mothers' disempowerment in patriarchal motherhood, offers many strategies for the promotion of feminist mothering, including combining motherhood with paid employment, insisting that fathers be involved in childcare, engaging in activism, and creating a life outside of motherhood. Commenting on Gordon's study, maternal scholar Ericka Horwitz observes: "Her [Gordon's] findings suggest that mothers can hold beliefs that are not in agreement with those promoted by the dominant discourses on motherhood. Gordon alerts us to the possibility that the process of resistance entails making different choices about how one wants to practice mothering" (44). Gordon, Glickman, and Green look specifically at mothers who identify as feminists, whereas Horwitz in her research examines empowered mothering: "the experiences of women who believe they were resisting the dominant discourse of mothering ... [but] who may or may not see themselves as feminist" (44-45). Empowered mothering signifies a general resistance to patriarchal motherhood; feminist mothering, however, refers to a particular style of empowered mothering in which this resistance is developed from and expressed through a feminist identification or consciousness.

Feminist mothering scholarship refuses the patriarchal profile and script of motherhood by challenging and changing the various ways patriarchal motherhood becomes oppressive to women. In *Of Woman Born*, Rich writes, "We do not think of the power stolen from us and the power withheld from us in the name of the institution of motherhood" (275). "The idea of maternal power has been domesticated," Rich continues, "in transfiguring and enslaving woman, the womb—the ultimate source of the power—has historically been turned against us and itself made into a source of powerlessness" (68). Rich argues that the institution of motherhood must be abolished so that the "potential relationship of woman to her powers of reproduction, and to children" can be realized (13). The central aim of feminist mothering is to reclaim power for mothers as well as to imagine and implement a mode of mothering that mitigates the many ways that patriarchal motherhood, both discursively and materially, regulates and restrains mothers and their mothering. A feminist mother seeks the eradication of motherhood as she recognizes that it is a patriarchal institution, in which gender inequality, or more specifically the oppression of women, is enforced, maintained, and perpetuated. Feminist mothering is, thus, primarily concerned with the empowerment of mothers. A theory of feminist mothering, therefore, begins with recognition that a mother must live her life and practice mothering from a position of agency, authority, authenticity, autonomy, and activism. A feminist standpoint on mothering affords a woman a life, a purpose, and an identity outside and beyond motherhood, and it does not limit childrearing to the biological mother. Likewise, from this standpoint, a woman's race, age, sexuality, or marital status does not determine her capacity to mother. A feminist theory on motherhood also foregrounds maternal power and confers value to mothering. Mothering from a feminist perspective and practice redefines motherwork as a social and political act. In contrast to patriarchal motherhood, which limits mothering to privatized care undertaken in the domestic sphere, feminist mothering is explicitly and profoundly political and social. Feminist mothering is also concerned with feminist practices of gender socialization and models of mother-child relations so as to raise a new generation of empowered daughters and empathetic sons. The achievement of antisexist childrearing, however, depends on the abolition of patriarchal motherhood. Mothers cannot facilitate changes in childrearing in an institution in which they have no power, as in the case with patriarchal motherhood. Antisexist childrearing necessitates motherhood itself being changed; it must become, to use Rich's terminology, "mothering." In other words, only when mothering becomes a site, a role, and an identity of power for women is feminist childrearing made possible. In dismantling patriarchal motherhood, mothers are invested with the needed agency and authority to create the desired feminist childrearing. Only then does antisexist childrearing become possible.

The above review reveals that the topic of feminist mothering has indeed become an established field of inquiry in motherhood studies, with many themes and topics examined as well as diverse strategies provided for the empowerment of mothers. However, as feminist scholars regard feminist mothering as essential for women's equality and autonomy as well as for the desired societal change in gender roles, their focus has been singularly Western—examining the critique of patriarchal motherhood and the creation of feminist mothering solely in a North American context, with some research from Australia and the UK. As well, although themes of feminist mothering have been identified and explored in the scholarship on African American and Indigenous mothering, they have been largely developed from a theoretical perspective and, thus, lack empirical corroboration or narrative consideration (Hill-Collins; Bell-Scott et al.; Hooks; Lorde; Walker; Lawson; Edwards; James; Wane; Thomas; Brant). I argue that this Western bias limits our understanding of the radical possibilities of feminist mothering and deters the formation of a truly transnational politic and practice for and about maternal empowerment. What is needed is research that foregrounds and amplifies how cultural location informs and mediates the manner in which patriarchal motherhood may be resisted and feminist mothering attained. As well, to fully understand and appreciate the transformative possibilities of maternal empowerment, we need to listen to the voices of actual mothers and their own lived perceptions and experiences of feminist mothering. Finally, we need to open up the theory and practice of feminist theory to the more expansive concept of feminist parenting so as to degender the revolutionary potential of transformative love and care.

Feminist Parenting: Perspectives from Africa and Beyond expands and, indeed, troubles contemporary theories and concepts of feminist parenting precisely in its foregrounding of diverse maternal subjectivities and in its consideration of the hitherto unexamined challenges and possibilities of feminist parenting. Some contributors (Nabaneh, Fofana, and Ka) reflect upon how their Islamic faith interfaces with their feminist ideology in their theory and practice of feminist parenting. Other contributors (Ghosal and Toure) consider how feminist mothering is practiced beyond the normative formations of the nuclear family. Foregrounding the politic, praxis, and pedagogy of feminist mothering first theorized by Green (discussed above), other contributors are attentive to how specific cultural contexts may constrain or compromise women's resistance to patriarchal motherhood and patriarchy more generally. Khan and Ndinga-Kanga, for example, consider how their outlaw identities and practices—being a feminist in Pakistan for Khan and being a queer feminist in South Africa for Ndinga-Kanga—make feminist resistance risky and perilous. The topic of single parenting is explored by several contributors in the collection with each contributor acutely aware as to how the possibilities and challenges of single parenting are determined by the culture in which it is practiced. Haas, for example, explores how her decision to adopt a child as a single young woman defied normative beliefs about parenting and adoption in her country of Uganda, whereas Adegbeye reflects upon how becoming a mother outside of marriage in Nigeria resulted in her being alienated from her family. The chapters authored by men similarly nuance the emergent scholarship on feminism, men, and fathering in their careful consideration of how gender socialization is culturally enacted and, simultaneously, how it may be resisted. Sene, a Senegalese man, describes how in being a father to a daughter, he became a feminist ally whereas Ngwena, a young Kenyan man, describes how he came to feminism through the presence of strong women in his life, including his single mother. Overall, each chapter in its own way identifies the limitations of Western feminism to address the needs of women from the Global South. Jael Stillman, for example, advocates for a global feminism and argues that "for feminism to be relevant in a Third World context, it has to address the legacy of colonialism that undergirds the structures of global context." (chapter four; p. 62) This collection is indeed a relevant and timely contribution to the scholarship on feminist parenting.

This collection opens up new pathways to both enhance and problematize the current scholarship by providing lived accounts of the challenges and possibilities of feminist parenting across cultures and maternal identities. In using the word new I am not suggesting that these pathways are new to the feminist parents of this collection but rather they are new to the Western trajectories and topographies of feminist mothering. The many and diverse voices of feminist mothers in this collection, including those of male allies, confirm that feminist parenting as a politic and practice is, indeed, more multifaceted and nuanced than Western theory would suggest. Exploring feminist parenting across various countries—Ghana, India, Senegal, the Gambia, Ecuador, the United Kingdom, the United States, Ethiopia, Germany, Pakistan, South Africa, Uganda, Nigeria, France, India, and Kenya—and from a multitude of standpoints, including single, queer, young, rural, non-custodial, bereaved, activist, community mothers, the collection reveals that the journeys of feminist parenting are neither uniform nor straightforward; there are struggles and successes. Moreover, the collection in its multiplicity of perspectives and locations confirms and affirms that feminist parenting is indisputably and indelibly transnational in both its theory and practice. Indeed, in foregrounding the many and diverse trajectories and topographies of feminist parenting, *Feminist Parenting: Perspectives from Africa and Beyond* moves us beyond established routes to chart new pathways of feminist parenting to extend, expand, and enhance its transformative power.

Work Cited

Bell-Scott, Patricia, et al., eds. *Double Stitch: Black Women Write about Mothers and Daughters*. Harper Perennial, 1993.

Brant, Jennifer. "Aboriginal Mothering: Honouring the Past, Nurturing the Future." *Mothers, Mothering and Motherhood across Cultural Difference*, edited by Andrea O'Reilly, Demeter Press, 2014, pp. 41-64.

Butterfield, Elizabeth. "Maternal Authenticity." *Encyclopedia of Motherhood*, edited by Andrea O'Reilly. Sage Press, 2010, pp. 700-1.

Copper, Baba. "The Radical Potential in Lesbian Mothering of Daughters." *Maternal Theory: Essential Readings*, edited by Andrea O'Reilly, Demeter Press, 2007, pp. 186-93.

Douglas, Susan J., and Meredith Michaels. *The Mommy Myth: The Idealization of Motherhood and How It Has Undermined Women*. Free Press, 2004.

Edwards, Arlene E. "Community Mothering: The Relationship between Mothering and the Community Work of Black Women." *Mother Outlaws: Theories and Practices of Empowered Mothering*, edited by Andrea O'Reilly, Women's Press, 2004, pp. 203-12.

Glickman, Rose L. *Daughters of Feminists: Young Women with Feminist Mothers Talk about Their Lives*. St. Martin's Press, 1993.

Gordon, Tuula. *Feminist Mothers*. New York University Press, 1990.

Gore, Ariel, and Bee Lavender. *Breeder: Real Life Stories from the New Generation of Mothers.* Seal Press, 2001.

Green, Fiona. *Feminist Mothering in Theory and Practice: 1985–1995.* The Edwin Mellin Press, 2009.

Hill-Collins, Patricia. *Black Feminist Thought: Knowledge, Consciousness, and the Politics of Empowerment.* 2nd ed. Routledge, 2000.

Hill, Shirley A. "African American Mothers: Victimized, Vilified, Valorized." *Feminist Mothering*, edited by Andrea O'Reilly, SUNY Press, 2008, pp. 107-22.

hooks, bell. "Homeplace: A Site of Resistance." *Maternal Theory: Essential Readings*, edited by Andrea O'Reilly. Demeter Press, 2007, pp. 266-73.

hooks, bell. *Talking Feminist, Talking Black.* South Ends Press, 1989.

Horwitz, Erika. "Resistance as a Site of Empowerment: The Journey Away From Maternal Sacrifice." *Mother Outlaws: Theories and Practices of Empowered Mothering*, edited by Andrea O'Reilly, Women's Press, 2004, pp. 43-58.

Horwitz, Erika. *Through the Maze of Motherhood: Empowered Mothers Speak.* Demeter Press, 2011.

James, Stanlie M. "Mothering: A Possible Black Feminist Link to Social Transformation." *Theorizing Black Feminisms: The Visionary Pragmatism of Black Women*, edited by Stanlie James and A.P. Busia, Routledge Press, 1999, pp. 44-54.

Lawson, Erica. "Black Women's Mothering in a Historical and Contemporary Perspective: Understanding the Past, Foraging the Future." *Mother Outlaws: Theories and Practices of Empowered Mothering*, edited by Andrea O'Reilly, Women's Press, 2004, pp. 193-202.

Lorde, Audre. "Man Child: A Black Feminist's Response." *Maternal Theory: Essential Readings*, edited by Andrea O'Reilly, Demeter Press, 2007, pp. 157-62.

Nathanson, Janice. "Maternal Activism: How Feminist is It?" *Feminist Mothering*, edited by Andrea O'Reilly, SUNY Press, 2008, pp. 243-56.

O'Brien-Hallstein, Lynn. "Maternal Agency." *Encyclopedia of Motherhood*, edited by Andrea O'Reilly, Sage Press, 2010, pp. 697-99.

O'Reilly, Andrea. "Between the Baby and the Bathwater: Some Thoughts on a Mother Centered Theory and Practice of Feminist Mothering." *Journal of the Association for Research on Mothering*, vol. 8, no. 1-2, 2006, pp. 323-30.

O'Reilly, Andrea. *Feminist Mothering*. SUNY Press, 2008.

O'Reilly, Andrea. *Matricentric Feminism: Theory, Activism and Practice.* Demeter Press, 2016.

O'Reilly, Andrea. *Rocking the Cradle: Thoughts on Motherhood, Feminism, and the Possibility of Empowered Mothering.* Demeter Press, 2006.

Powell, Pegeen Reichert. "Balancing Act: Discourses of Feminism, Motherhood and Activism." *Feminist Mothering*, edited by Andrea O'Reilly, SUNY Press, 2008, pp. 257-72.

Reddy, Maureen. *Everyday Acts against Racism*. Seal Press, 1996.

Reddy, Maureen, et al., eds. *Mother Journeys: Feminists Write about Mothering.* Spinsters Ink, 1994.

Rich, Adrienne. *Of Woman Born: Motherhood as Experience and Institution.* W.W. Norton, 1976.

Ruddick, Sara. *Maternal Thinking: Toward a Politics of Peace*. Beacon Press, 1989.

Stadtman Tucker, Judith. "Rocking the Boat: Feminism and the Ideological Grounding to the Twenty-First Mothers' Movement." *Feminist Mothering*, edited by Andrea O'Reilly, SUNY Press, 2008, pp. 205-18.

Thomas, Wanda Bernard, and Candance Bernard. "Passing the Torch: A Mother and Daughter Reflect on their Experiences Across Generations." *Canadian Women's Studies Journal/cahier de la femme*, vol. 18, no. 2-3, 1998, pp. 46-50.

Walker, Alice. *In Search of Our Mothers' Gardens: Womanist Prose.* Harcourt Brace Jovanovich, Publishers, 1984.

Wane, Njoki Nathani. "Reflections on the Mutuality of Mothering: Women, Children and Families." *Mother Outlaws: Theories and Practices of Empowered Mothering*, edited by Andrea O'Reilly, Women's Press, 2004, pp. 229-39.

Notes on Contributors

OluTimehin Adegbeye is a queer feminist nonfiction writer with a deep commitment to social justice, revolutionary love, and uninhibited dancing. In 2019, she won the Gerald Kraak prize for her essay, "Mothers and Men." Her TED Talk, "Who Belongs in a City?" was selected by TED as one of the most notable talks of 2017. She lives with her daughter in Nigeria.

Elena Damma balances her passion for humanity and the arts with her work for an international scientific institute. Despite an unexpected turn in her personal life, having a daughter has been an incredibly beautiful journey for her. Beyond that, she does not plan for the future, but she hopes that it will be filled with reflection, laughter, as well as good food, reads, and conversation with people with whom she feels she belongs.

Rama Salla Dieng, PhD, is a Senegalese scholar and writer. She is a Lecturer at the Centre of African Studies, University of Edinburgh, and a Research Associate of the Centre for Research on Families and Relationships of the same university. Rama is the Programme Director for the MSc Africa and International Development and her research focuses on African feminisms, feminist political economy, agrarian studies and gender and development in Africa. She currently serves on the Council of Development Studies Association UK, and convenes the Decolonising Development Study Group. Between 2010 and 2015, she worked at the Policy Research Division of the United Nations Economic Commission for Africa's Institute for Economic Development and Planning (IDEP) in Senegal. Rama has published a novel *La Dernière Lettre* with Présence Africaine in 2008. She has contributed to an edited volume by Gender Links on Polygamy: At the heart of the Matter (2009), and an edited volume on Democracy and Development:

Perspectives of Young African Researchers (2013) published by l'Harmattan. She holds a PhD and a MSc in International Development from SOAS, University of London and a Master in International Cooperation from Sciences Po Bordeaux, France.

Ousmane Diop worked for the British Council for over six years and then for the houses of parliament on a variety of projects. He met his partner in Senegal, which he left in 2008 to join her in London. Ousmane is passionate about politics and holds an MRes in public policy and management from Birkbeck University. He enjoys photography, football, and fixing things. And more than anything, he loves good discussions about the state of the world over some good food.

Elisabeth teaches and works on development projects and gender. Her rural upbringing in Germany in the 1970s immersed her in the pacifist movement, where feminism and ecology appeared as obvious allies. She moved to France in the early nineties. With her partner, she has brought up three daughters, trying to balance her feminist and ecologist aspirations.

Malaika Eyoh is a third-year student at the University of Toronto studying politics and African studies. She also studied at the University of Witwatersrand and was based there when she wrote this piece.

Joanna Grace Farmer, founder of Building Community Capacity (BCC), centres her work around increasing access to information and resources in order to strengthen and empower children, families, and communities, especially those most in need. BCC's areas of focus include political engagement; equitable community development, affordable housing, and quality education; culturally competent mental health systems; genealogy research; transformative pedagogy; and team building.

Kula Fofana is enrolled in a full-time graduate program at the School of Oriental and African Studies of the University of London. Prior to that, she served the Liberian government as assistant minister for youth development; cochaired Liberia's Vision 2030, and headed the Ministry of Gender, Children and Social Protection Adolescent Girls Division. For the most part, her longest career before government portfolios was in civil society organizations, working for young women and girls and vulnerable populations. With a BA in mass

Deepest appreciation to
Demeter's monthly Donors

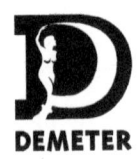

DEMETER

Daughters
Naomi McPherson
Linda Hunter
Muna Saleh
Summer Cunningham
Rebecca Bromwich
Tatjana Takseva
Kerri Kearney
Debbie Byrd
Laurie Kruk
Fionna Green
Tanya Cassidy
Vicki Noble
Bridget Boland

Sisters
Kirsten Goa
Amber Kinser
Nicole Willey
Regina Edwards